AF531370

Public Relations
and
Integrated Communications

Published by
Lotus Press

Public Relations and Integrated Communications

Stuart M. Levy

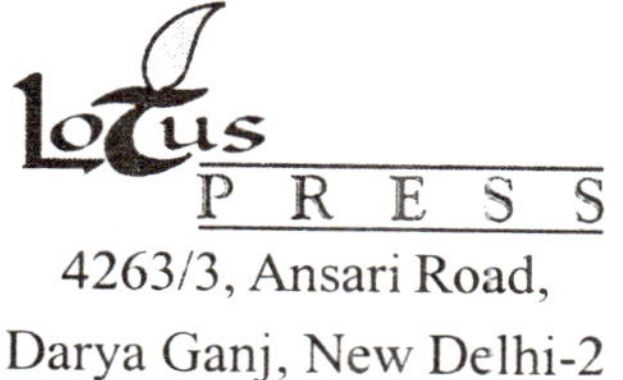

4263/3, Ansari Road,
Darya Ganj, New Delhi-2

LOTUS PRESS
4263/3, Ansari Road, Darya Ganj, New Delhi-110002
Ph: 30903912, 23290047, E-mail: lotus_press@sify.com

Public Relations and Integrated Communications

ISBN 81-8382-035-2

Published by: Lotus Press, New Delhi-110002
Lasertypeset by: Reliable Infomedia, New Delhi-110009
Printed at: Gyan Sagar, New Delhi

PREFACE

Public relations is the art and science of building relationships between an organization and its key audiences. Corporations use marketing public relations to convey information about the products they manufacture or services they provide to potential customers to support their direct sales efforts. Non-profit organisations, including schools and universities, hospitals, and social service agencies, use public relations in support of fund-raising programmes and staff recruiting, and to increase patronage of their services. Politicians use public relations to attract votes and raise money, and, when successful at the ballot box, to promote and defend their service in office, with an eye to the next election or, at career's end, to their legacy.

As the media grows more ruthless, the role of public relations has become increasingly complex and critical. Savvy business people know that how a company conveys and maintains its image has never been more important or more challenging.

This book is meant for media relations professionals, government public relations officers, practising public relations, satellite media tour, issues management system, public relations objectives, public relations practitioners, integrated marketing communications, public relations planning, public relations research, video news release and corporate communicators.

Editor

CONTENTS

1

INTRODUCTION

Public relations (PR) is the means and industry of influencing public opinion towards an organisation and its products or services. Public relations clients include political parties, ruling or otherwise. PR is distinct from advertising as it is generally not aimed at selling a particular product from a particular business, and, for further comparison, propaganda, sometimes carried out for political purposes by governments. Many of the same PR techniques may be employed in all these areas. Within the industry, those involved in marketing may consider public relations a subfield of marketing; those involved in PR may disagree.

Precursors to public relations can be found in publicists who specialised in promoting circuses, theatrical performances, and other public spectacles. Later, most PR practitioners were and are still recruited from the ranks of journalism. Journalists concerned with ethics question former colleagues for using their inside understanding of news media, helping clients receive favorable media coverage. Highly paid PR positions remain a popular career change choice for many journalists. PR historians say the first PR firm, the Publicity Bureau, was established in 1900 by former newspapermen, with Harvard University as its first client. The First World War also helped stimulate the development of public relations as a profession.

Many of the first PR professionals, including Ivy Lee, Edward Bernays, and Carl Byoir, got their start with the Committee for Public Information, which organised publicity on behalf of U.S. objectives during World War I. Some historians regard Ivy Lee as the first real practitioner of public relations, but Edward Bernays is generally regarded today as the profession's founder. Ivy Lee, who has been credited with developing the modern news release (also called a "press release"), espoused a philosophy consistent with what has sometimes been called the "two-way street" approach to public relations, in which PR consists of helping clients listen as well as communicate messages to their publics.

In the words of the Public Relations Society of America (PRSA), "Public relations helps an organisation and its publics adapt mutually to each other." In practice, however, Lee often engaged in one-way propagandising on behalf of clients despised by the public, including robber baron John D. Rockefeller. Bernays was the profession's first theorist. A nephew of Sigmund Freud, Bernays drew many of his ideas from Freud's theories about the irrational, unconscious motives that shape human behavior. Bernays authored several books, including Crystallising Public Opinion, Propaganda, and The Engineering of Consent. Bernays saw public relations as an "applied social science" that uses insights from psychology, sociology, and other disciplines to scientifically manage and manipulate the thinking and behavior of an irrational and "herdlike" public.

"The conscious and intelligent manipulation of the organised habits and opinions of the masses is an important element in democratic society," he wrote in Propaganda. "Those who manipulate this unseen mechanism of society constitute an invisible government which is the true ruling power of our country." One of Bernays' early clients was the tobacco industry. In 1929, he orchestrated a legendary publicity stunt aimed at persuading women to take up cigarette smoking, which was then considered unfeminine and inappropriate for women with any social standing. To counter this image, Bernays arranged for New York City débutantes to march in that year's Easter Day Parade, defiantly smoking cigarettes as a statement of rebellion against the norms of a male-dominated society.

Photographs of what Bernays dubbed the "Torches of Liberty Brigade" were sent to newspapers, convincing many women to equate smoking with women's rights. Some women went so far as to demand membership in all-male smoking clubs, a highly controversial act at the time.

PR may target different audiences with different messages to achieve an overall goal. Public Relations sets out to effect widespread opinion and behavior changes. Modern public relations uses a variety of techniques including opinion polling and focus groups to evaluate public opinion, combined with a variety of high-tech techniques for distributing information on behalf of their clients, including satellite feeds, the Internet, broadcast faxes, and database-driven phone banks to recruit supporters for a client's cause. According to the PRSA,

"Examples of the knowledge that may be required in the professional practice of public relations include communication arts, psychology, social psychology, sociology, political science, economics, and the principles of management and ethics. Technical knowledge and skills are required for opinion research, public issues analysis, media relations, direct mail, institutional advertising, publications, film/video productions, special events, speeches, and presentations."

Although public relations professionals are stereotypically seen as corporate servants, the reality is that almost any organisation that has a stake in how it is portrayed in the media employs at least one PR manager. Large organisations may even have dedicated communications departments. Government agencies, trade associations, and other nonprofit organisations commonly carry out PR activities. Public relations should be seen as a management function in any organisation. An effective communication, or public relations, plan for an organisation is developed to communicate to an audience (whether internal or external publics) in such a way the message coincides with organisational goals and seeks to benefit mutual interests whenever possible.

As industry consolidation becomes more prevalent, many organisations and individuals are choosing to retain "boutique" firms as opposed to so-called "global" communications firms. These smaller firms typically specialise in only a couple of practice areas and thus, often have a greater understanding of their client's business. And because they deal with certain journalists with greater frequency, specialty firms often have stronger media contacts in the areas that matter most to their clients. Added benefits of smaller, specialty firms include more personal attention and accountability and as well, cost savings. This is not to say that smaller is always better, but there is a growing consensus that specialty firms offer more than once considered.

A number of specialties exist within the field of public relations, including:

— crisis management

— reputation management

— issue management

— investor relations and labor relations

— grassroots PR (sometimes referred to as astroturf PR).

Public relations involves the management and distribution of information to enable an organisation's target audiences to understand its policies and programmes.

The role of public relations is to:

a) place a subject on the public agenda;
b) garner public support and endorsement of a person, product, organisation or idea;
c) extend advertising campaigns; and
d) deliver complex information and messages (which can not be delivered by an advertisement).

Public relations practice is broader than media relations and/or publicity generation. In reality, the activities of public relations practice include:

— *Issues management*: involves proactive systematic identification of issues of potential concern to an organisation and development of a system to respond to them.

— *Crisis management*: involves reactive systematic identification of issues and an appropriate response mechanism for unanticipated situations.

— *Media relations*: involves dealing with the media in seeking publicity for, or responding to, media interest in an organisation, person, product or idea.

— *Merchandising support*: the packaging of a product, an idea or person.

— *Event management*: involves planning activities or staging events which will attract media attention to a person, organisation, idea or product. A launch is a typical example.

— *Promotion*: attempts to garner the support and endorsement for a person, product, organisation or idea. Although promotion incorporates special events - which could be called event management - promotion goes into other areas, for example, storylines about the specific issue in soap operas, competitions or documentaries.

— *Public affairs*: a highly specialised kind of public relations which involves community and government relations - which is dealing with officials within the community and working with legislative groups and various pressure groups such as consumers.

— *Publicity*: involves disseminating purposefully planned and executed messages through selected media, without payment to the media, to further the particular interest of an organisation or person. Publicity is a tool used by public relations practitioners - it is not public relations in itself.

— *Sponsorship*: is a contractual agreement between two parties whereby benefits such as money or services in kind are traded for promotional opportunities offered by a campaign or event, for example, naming rights, brand exposure, corporate recognition, or endorsements.

METHODS, TOOLS AND TACTICS

The most fundamental rule in public communications is to know who one's audience is, and to tailor every message to appeal to that audience. An "audience" can be a general, nationwide or worldwide audience, but it is more often a segment of a population. Marketers often refer to economy-driven "demographics," such as "white males 18-49," but in public relations an audience is more fluid, being whoever the client wants to reach. For example, recent political audiences include "soccer moms" and "NASCAR dads." In addition to audiences, there are usually stakeholders, literally people who have a "stake" in a given issue.

All audiences are stakeholders (or presumptive stakeholders), but not all stakeholders are audiences. For example, a charity commissions a PR agency to create an advertising campaign to raise money to find a cure for a disease. The charity and the people with the disease are stakeholders, but the audience is anyone who is likely to donate money. Sometimes the interests of differing audiences and stakeholders common to a PR effort necessitate the creation of several distinct but still complementary messages. This is not always easy to do, and sometimes - especially in politics - a spokesperson or client says something to one audience that angers another audience or group of stakeholders.

Press Conference

A press conference consists of someone speaking to the media at a predetermined time and place. Press conferences usually take place in a public or quasi-public place. Press conferences provide an excellent opportunity for speakers to control information and who gets it; depending on the circumstances, speakers may hand-pick the journalists they invite to the conference instead of making themselves available to any journalist who wishes to attend. It is also assumed that the speaker will answer journalists' questions at a press conference, although they are of course not obliged to. However, someone who holds several press conferences on a topic (especially a scandal) will be asked questions by the press, regardless of whether they indicate they will entertain them, and the more conferences the person holds, the more aggressive the questioning may become.

Therefore, it is in a speaker's interest to answer journalists' questions at a press conference to avoid appearing as if they have something to hide. But questions from reporters - especially hostile reporters - detracts from the control a speaker has over the information they give out. For even more control, but less interactivity, a person may choose to issue a press release.

Press Releases

Press release format: The typical press release announces that the statement is "FOR IMMEDIATE RELEASE" across the top (some may instead be embargoed until a certain date), and lists the issuing organisation's media contacts directly below. The media contacts are the people that the release's issuer wants to make available to the media; for example, a press release about new scientific study will typically list the study's lead scientist as its media contact. The bottom of each release is usually marked with ### or -30- to signify the end of the text.

A press release is simply a written statement distributed to the media. It is a fundamental tool of PR work. Press releases are usually sent via a newswire service (such as PR Newswire or Business Wire) to media outlets, where journalists may pick them up and use them as they see fit. Very often the information in a press release finds its way verbatim, or minimally altered, to print and broadcast reports. If a media outlet reports that "John Doe said in a statement today that...", the "statement" was almost always a press release.

The text of the press release is usually (but not always) written as a news story, with an eye-catching headline and an article written in standard journalistic inverted pyramid style. This style is effective for reaching harried, and often skeptical journalists who rarely read entire releases. It also makes it easy for journalists to lift entire passages from a release and insert them into their own article. While this practice is frowned upon in newsrooms, journalism is a deadline-driven industry, and it is not uncommon for reporters to occasionally copy or modify a line or two from a press release. PR practitioners, on the other hand, design releases to encourage as much "lifting" as possible, so in essence, the less professional a journalist is, the more successful the release is judged to be.

The only time that journalists may copy from a press release in good conscience is if the release provides a direct quote, as in: Senator Smith said, "This is the most fiscally irresponsible bill that the Congress has passed since the Buy Everyone A Mercedes Act." In this case, a journalist may copy the quote verbatim into his or her story, although most reporters prefer to try soliciting an individual quote from the speaker before filing their story. However, because press releases reflect their issuer's preferred interpretation or packaging of a story, journalists are often skeptical of their contents. Of course, the level of skepticism, if any, depends on what the story is and who's telling it. Newsrooms receive so many press releases that, unless it is a story that the media are already paying attention to, a press release alone isn't always enough to catch a journalist's attention. With the advent of modern media and new technology, press releases now have equivalents in these media - video news releases and audio news releases.

Other methods are the following:

— Publicity events or publicity stunts.

— The talk show circuit. A PR spokesperson (or his/her client) "does the circuit" by being interviewed on television and radio talk shows with audiences that the client wishes to reach.

— Books and other writings.

— After a PR practitioner has been working in the field for a while, he or she accumulates a list of contacts in the media and elsewhere in the public affairs sphere. This "Rolodex" becomes a prized asset, and job announcements sometimes even ask for candidates with an existing Rolodex, especially those in the media relations area of PR.

Politics and Civil Society

Political campaigns are peak times for defining one's opponents, though the process occurs continually. Organisations and other groups of people can be defined just as easily as candidates. In the 2004 US presidential campaign, George W. Bush defined John Kerry as a "flip-flopper," among other characterisations, which were widely reported and repeated by the media, particularly the conservative media. Similarly, George H.W. Bush characterised Michael Dukakis as weak on crime (the Willie Horton ad) and as hopelessly liberal. In 1996, President Bill Clinton seized upon opponent Bob Dole's promise to take America back to a simpler time, promising in contrast to "build a bridge to the 21st century." This painted Dole as a person who was somehow opposed to progress.

In the debate over abortion, pro-abortion rights groups defined their opponents by defining themselves instead: "pro-choice." Anti-abortion rights groups responded in kind, branding themselves "pro-life." Extrapolating their respective rhetorics, pro-choice groups refer to their opponents as "anti-choice," and pro-life groups refer to their opponents as "pro-abortion." More recently, opponents of same-sex marriage in the U.S. have declared that their opponents are not the gay couples suing for the right to marry in various state courts, but rather the judges who rule in their favor. They are now calling them "activist judges," implying that they impose their personal beliefs instead of objectively interpreting the law. This sidesteps the thorny issue of making millions of gay people an "enemy," and instead focuses attention on the much smaller judiciary, who all Americans can ostensibly agree should be prevented from being "activists" on the bench.

If a politician or organisation can use an apt phrase in relation to an issue, such as in interviews or news releases, the news media will often repeat it verbatim, thus furthering the message. "New Deal" became a description of President Franklin D. Roosevelt's anti-Depression economic plans, and "states' rights/state sovereignty" became near-code words for anti-civil rights legislation. Recent examples come almost solely from Republican politicians: "death tax" for estate tax, "racial preferences" for affirmative action, "faith-based" instead of religious, among others.

Entertainment and Celebrity

A famous saying goes "Any publicity is good publicity," and celebrities tend to be fans of this dictum. If a celebrity says or does something embarrassing, he or she will often turn it into a strength and make it part of his or her "image." Of course, this tactic is used just as much with favorable situations as much as with unfavorable ones. A current example involves the entertainer Jessica Simpson, who gained nationwide prominence when she wondered aloud on a reality show if "Chicken of the Sea"-brand tuna fish was actually chicken or tuna, garnering her a reputation for being slow-witted. But by the summer of 2004, she was being paid to endorse a brand of breath mints called "Liquid Ice."

In the product's television commercial, Simpson replicates her earlier confusion by debating whether the mint is really liquid or ice. So although she was previously ridiculed, she (and her advisers) turned her nationwide embarrassment into a lucrative endorsement deal. Top US entertainment publicists include Lizzie Grubman, Karen Ammond, and PMK Public Relations.

As Oscar Wilde is supposed to have said, the only thing worse than being talked about is not to be talked about at all. Many celebrities seem to take this truism to heart, because when their popularity (and income) wane, they take on new projects that attract media attention. Considering that a celebrity's celebrity is a brand unto itself, many celebrities are under constant pressure to "reinvent" themselves, as a prophylactic against obscurity. A current trend among American celebrities is the transformation of musicians, comedians, and almost every other sort of performer into children's book authors. Madonna, Jay Leno, Billy Crystal, and several other celebrities have recently written children's books, accompanied by much media coverage.

A more traditional way of branching out is the celebrity restaurant. This is especially common among professional athletes, whose time in the spotlight is often limited by the physical demands of their jobs. Basketball player Michael Jordan opened a restaurant in Chicago, Illinois, and singer Britney Spears opened an ill-fated eatery in New York which closed a few months later.

Male celebrities like Tim Robbins, Sean Penn and Charlton Heston seem to gravitate toward politics, although some female celebrities, such as Susan Sarandon and Barbra Streisand, also become strong political voices. Younger female celebrities on the other hand are often drawn into the fashion world. Hotel heiress Paris Hilton recently announced that she was starting her own line of jewelry, and Jennifer Lopez has started a line of clothing. And fading star Elizabeth Taylor launched a fragrance called "White Diamonds" several years ago, bringing renewed interest from the media.

ETHICAL AND SOCIAL ISSUES

Many of the techniques used by PR firms are drawn from the institutions and practices of democracy itself. Persuasion, advocacy, and education are instruments through which individuals and organisations are entitled to express themselves in a free society, and many public relations practitioners are engaged in practices that are widely considered as beneficial, such as publicising scientific research, promoting charities, raising awareness of public health concerns and other issues in civil society. One of the most controversial practices in public relations is the use of front groups—organisations that purport to serve a public cause while actually serving the interests of a client whose sponsorship may be obscured or concealed.

The creation of front groups is an example of what PR practitioners sometimes term the third party tech—the art of "putting your words in someone else's mouth." PR Watch, a nonprofit organisation that monitors deceptive PR activities, has published numerous examples of this technique in practice. Current issues in ethical and social arenas have been brought to the attention of people from all stratas of the population when it was determined that more than one journalist with a platform had received money from a Public Relations firm for espousing a certain point of view.

COMMUNICATION

Public information, public relations, communications: international institutions seem to use these words interchangeably, moving from one to another and back again as successive waves of "reform" come and go. In publicly financed institutions such as UNESCO, public information constitutes an organic function. Keeping the public abreast of developments and debates in the worlds of education, science, culture, social sciences and communication is one of the reasons for which UNESCO exists. Doing it and doing it right is not only clever.

It is an essential part of UNESCO's mandate. Reflecting UNESCO's broad and diverse areas of responsibility, its Bureau of Public Information seeks to draw attention to a wide range of activities. It relies to do so on the research and expertise of colleagues throughout the house to spotlight important social and ethical issues, to nurture the democratic debate—with facts, figures and analysis— and to press for change where change is required.

Public information is, in other words, one of the organisation's principal weapons in the pursuit of its fundamental objectives. A recipe for failure There is enormous, probably limitless interest in the public and media for new data and insights on issues like cloning and bioethics in general, the state of oceans and coastlines, the sharing of fresh water resources, the education of girls, the digital divide, freedom of the press, teachers' salaries and working conditions, endangered cultural treasures—the list is a long one—that are UNESCO's bread and butter. This demand affords UNESCO with constantly renewed opportunities to advertise its concerns and programmes and to irrigate public opinion with its values.

In all cases however, what the public and media hunger for is information about the issue itself, not about the institution—and even less about its servants or component units. Failing to recognise this as self-evident is a recipe for failure. Results periodically achieved—massive, worldwide media coverage of UNESCO's reports and initiatives on EFA, trafficking of cultural goods, underwater heritage, disappearing languages, for example—have underlined the enormous appeal of the research and analysis for which UNESCO is uniquely qualified. More, better and more frequent reports are needed to meet that demand—and to put UNESCO back in the news.

A challenge to complacency Addressing as it must complex, often painful social realities, public information emanating from United Nations agencies cannot please all of the people all of the time. Genuine information is, by definition, a challenge to complacency which may at times lead to controversy and elicit protests. Seeking at all costs to avoid such developments is incompatible with the public information function. While there can be no place for gratuitous provocation, it must be accepted that no one has ever produced an omelette—in this case achieving influence over public opinion—without breaking some eggs. Public information's essential currency is credibility in the eyes of the media.

International organisations know, by painful experience, that this is not a given. Achieving and maintaining media credibility is above all an exercise in transparency which should be undertaken on the understanding that the reputation of international organisations must and will ultimately rest on the quality and relevance of their "real world" contribution. Empty posturing In the private sector as in politics, public relations are more often than not a question of putting one's best foot forward. Success is never guaranteed. Businesses and politicians are expected to have public relation strategies, but to describe their pronouncements as "PR" is not a compliment. In plain English it means rubbish, or something ruder. Taxpayer financed institutions cannot afford risks of this kind. They look especially bad when suspected of self-promotion or empty posturing.

Public relations for organisations like UNESCO should mean one thing only: exchanging information and developing working relations with different target audiences - constituents, parliamentarians, international organisations, provincial and municipal authorities, civic groups, NGOs, academic institutions, religious organisations, private enterprises—using language and supports appropriate to each. Public relations are, first and foremost, about dialogue. Their purpose is to build networks, to forge temporary or lasting alliances in order to achieve programme objectives: ratifications, project completions, policy changes, for example.

In some instances this dialogue should lead to operational partnerships, fund raising and other forms of collaboration. Public relations thereby represent an important entry point into the UN system for a wide range of potential partners. It stands to reason therefore that responsibility for engaging in public relations cannot be left to any single department. They must be conducted, as a matter of course and on a permanent basis, by directors and programme managers, indeed by all substantive officers at Headquarters and in the field.

Some will, on occasion, require material support. All rightfully expect policy guidance. Information kits and videos are welcome but not nearly as important as a regular internal flow of information on what must be clear, coherent and vigorously pursued objectives. So what about "communications"? What is left to "communications" is the heart of the matter, that which speaks louder than words: action. What will always matter more than what we say is what we do—or fail to do. Communications suffuse every aspect of the work of most UN bodies and agencies, including UNESCO. Standards, guidelines, codes of conduct, technical assistance: all are about sharing and spreading knowledge and values in order to affect change.

Successful communications imply transparency—public information—and outreach—public relations. But they, above all, require courage, conviction and initiative. Value-based endeavours are judged in the end, not by the noise they temporarily generate but by the difference they make in the lives of people. Nothing new there. What is perhaps new in a number of international organisations is a growing reliance on marketing techniques long on image-polishing but short on substance: glitter-studded media-oriented events, contrived "photo opportunities", glossy brochures. Some also seem more comfortable with slogans and sound bites, with ghostwritten "oped" pieces on consensual subjects than with the rougher give and take of press conferences and interviews with well-informed, aggressive reporters.

Those who claim expertise and leadership in social, economic or humanitarian matters, among others, must expect searching questions. These are inherent to democratic processes and should be welcomed as management tools. There is nothing wrong with gloss and glitter or with controlled appearances in the media provided these come in addition to—and not as a substitute for—genuine public information and public relations activities. One comes down to what you can afford. The other reflects—and projects—how significant you might be. There are no easy shortcuts in the battle for hearts and minds.

A communication strategy provides an essential framework for developing a comprehensive and integrated campaign. It is a plan which outlines the rationale for, and desired outcomes of, your proposed public information campaign. The strategy defines specific objectives to provide a framework within which to formulate strategies and against which to evaluate outcomes. In the development of the communication strategy, key decisions need to be made about:

— the range of integrated information activities to be implemented;
— what research the strategy is to be based on;
— how external consultants will be used;
— the roles and responsibilities of all key stakeholders in the strategy;
— the available budget;
— the timeline; and
— the evaluation plan.

The communication strategy should clearly articulate how all the various components of the campaign will be co-ordinated and managed to achieve its objectives most efficiently and effectively.

Importance of Communication Strategy

Before you write a brief for a public relations consultant, you need to write a communication strategy. Public relations is usually only one part of an integrated communication campaign and, as such, the role of the public relations activities needs to be clearly defined within the context of a communication strategy before a public relations brief can be written.

The PR brief is the foundation upon which the public relations consultant plans (and costs) their proposal. Therefore, a good brief is the key to receiving high quality, tightlyfocused proposals from consultants. A good PR brief will:

— provide enough detail about the programme/policy that it can be understood by someone who has no knowledge of the subject and key issues, and can be read as a stand alone document;
— explain the need for public relations and where it fits within the broader communication strategy;

— be supported and informed by research;
— clearly define the communication objectives;
— outline the tasks the successful consultant will perform;
— highlight any sensitivities which impact on the campaign;
— include a clear timeline for the campaign;
— outline any activities which will complement the campaign;
— describe the key stakeholders of the campaign and their role;
— clearly outline the tender task and the selection process; and
— facilitate evaluation of the campaign's success.

It is critical that the brief is comprehensible to consultants. Therefore, it is advisable to write the brief in plain English (ie avoid bureaucratic jargon or terminology too specific to particular programmes or policies). By writing a brief, you are seeking advice from professionals with specialist knowledge. Consultants are at the 'coalface' every day, and usually have a better knowledge of appropriate communication tactics than clients, so resist prescribing techniques which you think the consultant should use. Rather, give consultants the opportunity to demonstrate their knowledge and use it as a means of choosing between them. Using the consultants' expertise will facilitate proposal evaluation; you will then be able to compare the merits of a range of communication solutions and costings.

Aim of Communication

The aim should be a short statement of the desired outcome of the communication strategy. For example to increase the level of full age appropriate childhood immunisation coverage by creating a climate of acceptance and active support from both parents and service providers. Be realistic about what the strategy can achieve within the timeframe, budget and available resources. Remember, the most successful communication campaigns are underpinned by programme support strategies, which deliver the product or service that your communication strategy is addressing.

Clear, specific and measurable objectives are critical to the success of information activities: not only are they critical to the development of an appropriate public relations strategy, but they also form the basis of campaign evaluation. Therefore it is imperative that specific and measurable objectives are stated clearly in your brief. It is a common error to confuse objectives with tasks. When writing your brief be mindful of the following:

Tasks are what you/or your consultants do to achieve your objectives and commonly start with such words as "To develop..." "To implement..." for example:

— to develop an issues management strategy;

— to undertake a national launch of the campaign;

— to implement a three-month public relations campaign.

An objective is what you hope to achieve from your information activities (ie an outcome) and commonly start with such words as "To increase..." "To inform..." "To reinforce...". Research will assist you to develop realistic objectives. Your research will give you a greater understanding of current awareness and attitudes toward your subject matter and therefore provide a starting point for communication activity. When setting objectives you should:

— be realistic within the timeframe, budget and resources;

— ensure they are measurable;

— state what you aim to achieve in terms of the target audience:

Awareness, understanding and knowledge - most campaigns aim to increase awareness, understanding and knowledge of a government policy or programme. Awareness objectives relate to what you want your target audience to be informed or educated about.

Attitudes—favourable or unfavourable feelings about an issue, which are learned, and relatively enduring. It is assumed that changing attitudes will lead to an increase in the positive behaviours a campaign is promoting. Some campaigns aim to reinforce positive attitudes to ensure that positive behaviours are maintained; while others attempt to change negative attitudes. Attitude objectives are really a statement of how you want the target audience to feel about the issue.

Behaviours—are what you want the target audience to do as a result of being exposed to your campaign. Behaviours are the specific actions which you are encouraging members of the target audience to undertake. Some examples of objectives are:

To increase awareness with 18-40 year olds:

— of the immediate and longer term health effects of smoking;

— that every cigarette does physical damage; and

— that support for quitting smoking is available in various forms.

To generate/strengthen:

— personal relevance to the health messages of the campaign;

— a sense of the 'immediacy' of the health effects depicted in the campaign advertising; and

— the confidence of people aged 18-40 in their own ability to change their behaviour.

To increase intentions to:

— quit/attempt to quit smoking; and

— access available support services.

The public relations brief should not introduce objectives not outlined in the communication strategy. However, you might not necessarily wish to just replicate all the objectives found in the strategy. It may be that emphasis is placed on achieving some specific objectives in the public relations component of the campaign.

Target Audiences

Exactly who do you want to receive your message? Target audiences should be described in terms of:

— current behaviour.

— level of awareness.

— level of knowledge.

— preferred methods for receiving information.

— motivations/barriers to hearing and believing/accepting the information.

You should describe your target audiences in as much detail as possible. Broad descriptions such as the "general public" are less likely to lead to a successful campaign than a tightly defined target. The more thoroughly you understand your target audience/s, the higher the probability of success.

— *Primary Target Audience* —people/groups who will be directly affected by your message or need to be exposed to your message.

- *Secondary Target Audience*—people of less importance who you wish to receive the campaign messages, people who will also benefit from hearing the campaign messages or people who influence your target audience now or in the future: for example, general practitioners.
- *Stakeholders*—Other people/groups who might be directly or indirectly involved in, affected by or with a stake in your campaign.

The key messages should encapsulate the purpose of your communication activity in as few words as possible. Key messages do not need to be catchy. They are not the "slogan" or the "jingle" for your campaign or the actual words to be used as your message. There is time later, during campaign development, to mould your message into a form that is appropriate for your audience/s. Research indicates that the following types of messages are likely to be rejected:

- messages which are global in nature;
- messages which are a series of 'motherhood' statements;
- messages which are self congratulatory; or
- self-promotion without substance.

Effective key messages should include details of the programme or policy being promoted, the benefits of the initiative for the target audience, and a clear "call to action" outlining what the target audience should do as a result of receiving your messages. You should remember that public relations has the ability to deliver the more complex campaign messages and provide a level of detail which the advertising campaign can often not achieve. Careful consideration should be given to which messages are best suited to the public relations versus the advertising strategy.

Communication Mix

It is useful to outline the proposed components of the communication campaign to enable the consultant to understand the context within which the public relations activity will occur. For example, it is useful for the public relations consultant to know that a mass media advertising campaign is planned so that they can ensure synergy between the advertising and public relations strategies. If it is the intention of your department to carry out some of the public relations activities in-house, you must detail in the document exactly what the external public relations consultant will be responsible for and what the department will be managing.

Research: Research is used to guide the development, implementation and evaluation of information activities. It can, and does, prevent resource wastage by ensuring that the campaign is indeed necessary and appropriate for the target audience/s. You should include in your public relations brief details of any research conducted or proposed as part of the campaign, including:

— developmental research which has underpinned the strategy and messages;

— concept testing (to assist in selecting the advertising agency and refining creative concepts for advertising and products);

— benchmark and tracking the campaign (testing strategies, reporting on coverage and readership of your issue, checking recall); and

— evaluating the outcomes (checking for changes in target audience attitudes, knowledge, behaviour).

PR consultants should also be reminded to provide the department with details on how they propose to evaluate the effectiveness of the public relations strategy they are to implement.

Key Issues

Include details of any constraints on your information activities to give consultants the opportunity to consider issues that might impact on the campaign when preparing their proposals. Examples of issues for consideration include:

- subtleties of the communication task, such as "musts" and "must nots" in communicating the message and design;
- sensitive issues;
- the need to work in consultation with other consultants (eg market researcher, advertising agency, or a specialist non-English speaking background or indigenous Australians communications consultant);
- regional or geographical constraints;
- financial constraints;
- the need for materials to be approved by particular positions or by interest groups before release; and
- the approval process for campaign strategies and materials.

Tender Task

The consultant must be provided with specific details on what is expected of them as part of the tender process. This is distinct from the task required of the successful consultant which is defined in the final contract with the department. For example, as part of the tender process the consultant will be expected to:

- Develop a written proposal The proposal must include:
  - an outline of how the public relations strategy will be developed and implemented, if successful;

- — a rationale for the proposed strategic approach;
- — a proposed approach to launching the campaign;
- — strategic advice regarding other suitable publicity events;
- — details of an appropriate publicity programme including an issues management strategy;
- — an outline of a proposed approach to stakeholder management;
- — recommendations on and a rationale for information materials, if applicable;
- — a detailed timeline for implementing the strategy;
- — a detailed costing of services, including daily/weekly/hourly rates;
- — details of personnel who will be working on the strategy, clearly identifying roles and, if applicable, hourly rates;
- — details of similar projects worked on including the contact details of (three) referees;
- — an explanation of how the public relations strategy will be evaluated; and
- — details of reporting and invoicing formats and procedures.

— To assist the selection process, you should also detail in the brief that consultants must:

- — restrict the written proposal to 20 or fewer, A4 single-sided, numbered pages using a 12 point font size (excluding curriculum vitaes and company experience which would be less than 30 pages in an attachment to the main document);

  - provide an executive summary of no more than two pages;
  - provide a specific number of copies; and
  - include a table of contents.

Selection Criteria

State the criteria against which you are going to evaluate the consultants' proposals, which should be kept to a minimum to facilitate the selection process. The following selection criteria cover most requirements, although you can add others which you deem appropriate:

- Understanding of the issues.
- Clarity of the rationale for the proposed strategy.
- The quality of the proposed communication strategy
  - Are there clear links with the communication objectives?
  - Will the target audience/s be reached effectively by the proposed strategy?
  - Are the proposed communication vehicles appropriate for the campaign messages?
  - Do the proposed information materials clearly reflect the strategic approach?
- Innovation and creativity demonstrated within the strategy.
  - Will the proposed strategy have impact/cut through?
  - Are there ideas beyond standard public relations activities?
- Value for money:
  - an assessment of cost against perceived impact/ reach of the strategy.

— No conflict of interest.

— References from previous projects will be used to assess the consultant's ability on:

  — proven capacity to deliver projects on time and within budget; and

  — proven ability to work cooperatively with the department;

— relevant/related experience of the team of people who will work on the business.

Experience could be defined in terms of government experience, social marketing experience, subject matter experience or experience in developing and implementing similar communication activities, whichever is deemed to be most relevant to the campaign.

Task for Consultant

Clearly outline the tasks you expect the successful consultant to perform. The following examples cover a wide range of activities and may not always be relevant. For example:

The successful consultant will be required to:

— refine the winning proposal in consultation with the department;

— confirm the programme of activities/events to be developed as part of the strategy;

— develop and implement:

  — the final public detailed relations strategy as agreed with the department,

  — a launch strategy for the advertising campaign which includes liaising with the media to ensure maximum media coverage and the development of support materials,

    — a publicity programme to garner support for the campaign over a six month period,
    — a comprehensive issues management strategy,
    — a stakeholder management strategy.
— develop, produce and distribute supporting information materials;
— organise and manage publicity events;
— liaise with other consultants and key stakeholders as required;
— report regularly to the department on campaign progress;
— at the campaign's completion, submit a report containing:
    — copies of all media releases, fact sheets, invitation, running sheets, etc.,
    — print and electronic media clippings,
    — outline of other outcomes such as alliances, partnership activity, etc.,
    — summary of the strengths and weaknesses of the approach and recommendations for future public relations action,
    — budget summary,
    — an assessment of the outcomes and internal efficiencies,
    — on completion of the campaign provide all the artwork for creative material to the department.

SCHIZOPHRENIC WORLD OF PUBLIC RELATIONS

Public relations arose as a low-tech, person-to-person activity featuring stunts, events, and cozy relations with the press... all designed to attract attention. When it works, it still does. The underlying science mass communications, opinion leadership, cognitive dissonance, etc. does give public relations a patina of legitimacy. Accreditation of practitioners by the Public Relations Society of America is another gesture in that direction. But the business never strayed far from its roots. Get publicity, get attention. Spell the client's name right.

There's lots of room for real strategic planning and opinion sampling in any PR campaign. Online services like www.zoomerang.com, www.clicktomarket.com and www.inetsurveys.com are three URLs that belong on every PR person's short list of bookmarks. It's just that Media Map, PR Newswire, and Business Wire are going to be tapped a whole lot more in the course of a day's work. That doesn't mean the strategic intelligence of a Harold Burson, Pam Edstrom, or Regis Mc Kenna is outdated. But more than ever before, PR today is about publicity and media, and the consultants performing the worthy function of steering corporations into provident waters are just in a different business. In the dot-com, high tech, and B2Anyone worlds, PR might just as well mean Press Relations... if not Press Releases.

That could be one reason PR is headed for the couch. Aside from role confusion, the press we're trying to have relations with is fragmenting right along with the markets it serves.

FRAGMENTATION AND CROSS-DRESSING

Audiences are splintered into demographic shards, as prosperity and technology bring in their wake an explosion of interests and the time and money to pursue them. The gazillions of new print magazines, e-zines, and newsletters speak to our fragmented and passionate interests. This proliferation goes to the heart of the New

PR practice. The very concept of a "public" as an assemblage of people somehow constituting an audience vanished forever circa 1977 when the first Apple fell from the tree. From that time on, with increasing power, each citizen became an independent node in a communications network... and a publisher at will.

Under the velocity of change, the lines are blurring between traditional media and traditional PR. When Yahoo!, to some folks, is a slick magazine and The New York Times is something you read online in the morning, it's easy to see how online and offline media merge. Today, newspaper editors and online e-zine staff can pull their stories off PR wire services or press rooms on commercial web sites. Independent journalists and staff writers can do a good chunk of their research by going to online material produced by PR people. The forward slash separating Online/Offline, PR office/Newsroom is a permeable membrane. Although the basic paradigm continues unchanged, what has changed, forever, for both media and PR, is the traditional way of reaching those targets. And here is where PR comes into its own.

Only publicity has the option to work both these areas, go beyond the mythical segmented markets, beyond the niche pubs, into the never-never land of chat groups, discussion groups, list servs, and bulletin boards that never saw an ad dollar. PR people, by and large, are hired to get their clients publicity, not strategise. In the course of that work, they're clearly part of the expanding news media universe, integral to the gathering and dissemination of news.

2
CULTURE OF PUBLIC RELATIONS

Public relations is a multicultural field that entails an ongoing competition and cooperation among a finite number of cultural voices. Public relations not only contributes to cultural discourse; it also is a site of an ongoing cultural contest. Cultural theory in anthropology on the elementary relational structures proposes that "plural rationalities" organise social discourse. Cultural theory scholars labeled these different rationalities as "cultural biases."

A cultural bias is a worldview that cognitively supports a particular way of organising social relations. Each cultural bias has an accompanying set of preferred argument structures or cultural topoi. These CT organise discussions of value conflicts in society. These cultural biases also organise discourse about public relations. This competition of cultural voices appears in histories of public relations, accounts of professional practice, estimates of public relations's future trajectory, and normative prescriptions for public relations practice.

Think of culture as essentially a dialogue that allocates praise and blame. Then focus particularly on the blame. Cultural theory proposes that "culture" is an ecosystem inhabited by a finite number of ways of life. Culture emerges in the contentious conversation among the ways of life. A way of life consists of a preferred pattern of social relations and a cultural bias or set of shared values and beliefs about people and the natural world. These configurations of belief and social relations are "reciprocal, interacting and reinforcing. Adherence to a certain pattern of social relationships facilitates a distinctive way of looking at the world; adherence to a certain worldview legitimises a corresponding type of social relations".

A way of life is viable only as long as its cultural bias and its pattern of social relationships are compatible with each other. "A cultural voice" will refer to instances when the premises of a "cultural bias" are articulated in argument. In addition, a "cultural tribe" will refer to an "interpretive community" that shares a particular cultural bias. Cultural theory posits that the social construction of reality operates within set limits. There are only five enduring voices in the cultural competition; only fatalism, egalitarianism, hierarchy, autonomous individualism (AI), and competitive individualism are coherent enough to attain long term viability. A cultural bias is an internally consistent template that structures human relationships.

The core propositions of each cultural bias are also argument structures. A topos or topic structure is a general theme that can be used to develop persuasive arguments on a wide set of topics. A cultural topos is a systematic argument that reinforces a preferred pattern of social relationships. Each cultural voice has a core set of CT. The most fundamental arguments of each cultural voice are its assertions about "nature" and "human nature."

"That's the way the world is" or "That's the way people are" are final arguments put forward to quell further disputation. These beliefs about reality are associated with a supporting value imperative, a decision making principle, a justice principle, and an activity principle. The cultural voices fundamentally disagree with one another in their assertions about reality and the preferred structure of social relations.Thetopoi of the culturalvoices are ordered from left to right, from the simplest to the most complex, and in terms of the degree of strategic calculation required to sustain each type of social relations.

According to cultural theory, the five ways of life constitute a cultural ecosystem. Each way of life defines itself relative to its competitors, and each way of life competes for adherents. Each way of life waxes or wanes relative to the success that its topoi have in predicting, interpreting, and managing events. CT have great durability in cultural debates, even extending over several centuries. However, societal events can increase the allure of a cultural voice and diminish the potency of competing cultural voices. The terrorist attacks of September 11th strengthened the appeal of hierarchy (i.e., national security). Likewise, the collapse of Enron gave some new impetus to egalitarian initiatives like campaign finance reform. These gains have been at the expense of competitive individualist (CI) topoi that dominated discourse during the 1990s stock market boom.

Each cultural bias provides lenses for interpreting the world. Each way of life clearly sees what the other ways of life do not see. As with optical illusions, one can only see one thing at a time. To see differently, one must change lenses. Even when they agree on nouns and verbs, theways of life disagree on adjectives and adverbs. CIs celebrate the elegant efficiency in markets, but egalitarians bemoan wasteful and vindictive conspicuous consumption that markets enable.

Cultural theory proposes that each way of life is incomplete. "Eachway of life needs each of its rivals, either to make up for its deficiencies, or to exploit, or to define itselfagainst. To destroy the other (wayof life) is to murder the self". Away of life contains contradictions and pathologies. The ways of life compete and give form to culture. Each group develops its own set of compromises and social institutions. One voice may dominate discourse or two voices may form a dominant coalition. The remaining voices tend to be ignored or marginalised. Representative democracy is a coalition of cultures in which each voice is articulated somewhere in the differentiated institutions of representative democracy.

The cultural voices also collaborate. Two ways of life may share values and preferred means. They may support the same means for different reasons. Hierarchical advocates endorse school uniforms because they symbolise order, but egalitarian advocates embrace uniforms because they mute displays of social inequality. Cultural alliances and oppositions shift as historical circumstances change. For culture, there "is no final equilibrium point. Change is inherent in the different competencies and biases of different cultures". The hierarchical and egalitarian voices privilege the"common good" and disparage the opportunism of CIs and fatalists.

Egalitarians and individualists dislike the regimentation of hierarchical culture. Individualist and hierarchical voices defend the virtues of social inequality. The fatalist voice can be engaged in alliances of evasion and passive resistance. Fatalists may help individualists evade the organising impulses of hierarchy or passively assist hierarchy in preserving the status quo against the attacks of egalitarian reformers (i.e., the silent majority). Groups make difficult tradeoffs between the values embedded in the different cultural biases when they decide how to allocate scarce resources.

People experience anxiety, ambivalence, or outrage when they encounter such trade offs. For instance, an explicit discussion about how much an HMO should be required to spend on experimental medical treatments to save one individual's life causes us discomfort. Ordinarily, it is taboo to discuss such topics. To put a dollar value on human life offends our sensibilities.

CULTURAL THEORY AND PR

The CT perspective applies inanycontextwherepeople argueabouthowtheyshould organise their social relationships. This chapter employs a mix of discourse exemplars from public relations scholarship and professional publications that are available to public relations practitioners, as well as texts that criticise existing public relations institutionsandpractices. This approach emphasises the similarities and continuities between these different discourse genres. It also attempts to demonstrate that the CT framework has heuristic value: It is flexible and is applicable to discourse in each domain. A "rational text" uses a consistent set of topoi in its arguments.

However, some texts are internally inconsistent. A person may also believe that one domain (i.e., family life) fits one model, but that another domain (i.e., professional life) fits another model. The cultural voices also may agree on an ideological point. One sometimes must scrutinise arguments at a microlevel before the differences in underlying topoi become evident. The cultural voices also differ in how frequently they voice their concerns (e.g., fatalism). Mapping the subterranean features of argument also requires persistent attention to what remains unsaid.

Fatalist Voice

Fatalist culture is indifferent to disputes about the nature and obligations of public relations. The other cultural camps often disparage it. The fatalist tribe has low expectations for public relations as a whole. The fatalist voice is underrepresented in the discourse of professional associations. It seldom argues for or justifies the public relations function. Fatalist culture does not debate these issues because it perceives that public relations practitioners lack the power to order their situation. The factors that really affect public relations practice lay beyond practitioners' control (i.e., practitioners have an external locus of control). It offers few visions about the future of practice. Popular culture portrayals of fatalistic public relations depict public relations practitioners as obsequious, cynical, isolated, and unfulfilled.

The fatalist voice does not proselytise, but it is a voice of resistance. It speaks through inattention and excuses for inaction. It resists the exhortations to engage in programmatic action. When asked to support a programme to enhance the influence of public relations, the fatalist voice demurs because the proposed course of action is futile. Collective action will not make a significant difference. Closed ended survey questions seldom find the fatalist voice. However, in depth interviews and ethnographic observation can locate the fatalist voice as they probe practitioners' daily routines. It also becomes audible when outsiders appraise the discipline or when professionals confide about their disillusionment with the profession.

The fatalist voice also murmurs in despotic environments where practitioners perceive that unpredictable and capricious forces determine their fates. Celebrity public relations can be unpredictable and capricious. Publicity becomes an end in itself because it creates a celebrity premium that people are willing to pay for. However, "high visibility public relations" can be a high stakes, zero-sum game. The number of celebrities who can be created and maintained is rather finite and inelastic. "The more popular the sector, the more violently a person's celebrity status will fluctuate".

The fortunes of public relations promoters are driven by the fickle hand that determines who is hot and who is not. Even if celebrity public relations is successful, "the bad news is that publicists are often not included as an important player at the center of the visibility marketing process and are not financially rewarded at the same level as agents and managers". Indeed, the celebrity industry usually maintains a low profile. The ghost writer selectively sorts the facts of a life and creates a celebrity narrative that cannot publicly acknowledge the writer's contribution. The practitioner also must cope with the caprices of temperamental and neurotic celebrities. Hand holding is listed as one of the essential duties of the celebrity promoter because Celebrities often need reassurances and smiles of pseudo-intimacy.

...In a world in which it is very hard to evaluate with any precision what you're doing from day to day, a hand-holder supplies the important services of confidence building and ego maintenance. Moreover, creating a celebrity often creates an uncontrollable ego that "often grows into cockiness and arrogance". These tendencies often are cultivated by the "entourages of obsequious support personnel that surround the celebrity". Press agentry is often characterised as a residue of public relations practice from a different era that has been replaced by more productive and ethical public relations models. However, the chroniclers of "high visibility" declared that "celebrity worship and visibility seeking is in an explosive growth phase" that is spreading to all sectors of society. The fatalist voice emerges when "high visibility public relations" becomes a capricious zero-sum game.

The fatalist voice also appears in organisational public relations. Fatalist culture does not consider public relations to be a self-defining and self regulating system. Public relations is whatever top management says it is: a marginal organisational function that is not seated at the management roundtable. For instance, public relations may be subordinated to another organisational function. "PR has generally been treated as a marketing stepchild, an afterthought to more serious promotional planning". Within public relations research, a great deal of attention has been devoted to the study of the role that practitioners play within the organisation. The prevailing consensus is that most public relations practitioners work as technicians rather than as managers.

Unless a public relations department has at least one practitioner in a management role, the organisational influence of public relations will be minimised. In such environments, one might expect to find a fatalistic worldview. Leichty and Springston found that one of their five public relations role clusters endorsed aspects of the fatalistic voice. This group, which Leichty and Springston labeled as externals, thought the public relations department was peripheral to the communication flows in the organisation. They also thought the public relations department had little influence or power. This type of practitioner was usually the only full time public relations professional in the organisation. These practitioners had few opportunities for professional advancement within their organisations.

Some aspects of the fatalist voice also appear in the Personal Influence model of public relations. The personal influence modelwas defined as "a quid pro quo relationship between the public relations practitioner and strategically placed individuals such as government regulators, media persons and tax officials". The personal influence model is most likely to be employed in those nations in which public opinion is not well articulated in the media and where governmental officials are the most important audience for public relations messages.

Ehnographic account of public relations practice in Southern India found that public relations practitioners spent much of their time ingratiating themselves with powerful people. Practitioners provided small favors to gain personal favor and influence with powerful targets. Personal influence activities included "hospitality, giving gifts and brokering of influence, to build lasting friendships with strategically placed individuals with the aim of seeking favors in return". Most of the practitioners in his sample had public relations titles, but had little power to influence policy decisions in their organisations. Practitioners desired professional autonomy, but "most were reluctant to express this to their superiors because they thought that it would not make any difference".

The personal influence model was most likely in social contexts where there is a high deference to authority by subordinates and an intolerance of subordinates' viewpoints by superiors. Wherever low practitioner power and a capricious environment combine, personal influence will be cultivated as a means of coping. The fatalist view of public relations also appears in the disinterested assessments of outsiders. Peter Drucker, the renowned management consultant, opined:

> There is no public relations. There's publicity, promotion, advertising, but "relations" by definition are a two-way street. And the more important job and the more difficult is not to bring the business and execution to the outside but to bring the outside to terribly insulated people.

Drucker said public relations professionals fail to "tell the truth to management. Public relations people today don't do that because they are scared; because the people they work for don't like to hear what they don't want to hear".

Several developmental trajectories lead to a fatalistic view of public relations practice. One trajectory is the route of dashed expectations. A public relations professional may begin with an idealistic vision of how to practice public relations, but become cynical when these expectations are dashed.

A fatalistic viewpoint may develop when a practitioner encounters a chaotic environment that subverts normal public relations practice. Among high-tech companies, the quest to prop up a company's stock price often subverted public relations values. "When the stock price was up, all of us were heroes. When it was down, we were scapegoats". When the stock price starts to drop, "strategy for the most part, goes out the door. Forget setting goals and objectives and creating strategies and tactics. Forget the well thought out public relations plan that was created and approved at the beginning of the year". A practitioner may also embrace fatalist topoi after a precipitous career decline.

Fatalist culture shrugs off the insults of hierarchical culture, the malign neglect of individualist culture, and the proselytising fervor of egalitarian culture. It is better to face some of the unpleasant facts of public relations practice than it is to live in a fantasy world. It is best to persevere through the bad and to enjoy the good when it comes.

Egalitarian Voice

The egalitarian voice is a prophetic voice. It animates activists who seek to reduce social inequality. It has manifested itself in the abolitionists, the muckrakers, and many social movements in the 20th century. Although there is a fledgling in-house egalitarian public relations voice, this voice usually speaks from the periphery of public relations. It prefers to critique the establishment rather than to negotiate with it. Its voice animates conversations about the nature of public relations. Unflattering egalitarian characterisations of public relations are a feature of popular culture's depictions of public relations. Its stark characterisations of public relations practice energise the cultural voices of the dominant coalition to declare, "Public relations isn't at all like that".

Egalitarian critics of public relations accuse it of distorting communication and undermining the processes of participatory democracy. Stauber and Rampton accused public relations of having an antidemocratic bias. "This contemptuous attitude toward democracy is the heritage of Edward Bernays, the father philosopher of public relations who saw corporate 'engineering of consent' as away to eliminate the 'chaos' in democratic society". However, democracy is "chaotic, messy and unpredictable and most bothersome of all to PR practitioners, it often produces decisions that their clients are unable either to predict or control".

Authentic democracy "must be lived daily, its valueswoven into the fabric of society. ...Democracy is not like fast food. It can't be standardised, mass-produced, made predictable and convenient". Public relations threatens democracy because "raw money enables the PR industry to mobilise private detectives, attorneys, broadcast faxes, satellite feeds, sophisticated information systems and other expensive, high-tech resources to out-maneuver, overpower and outlast true citizen reformers". However, corporate public relations has an Achilles heel. "Today's opinion industry is a powerful giant, but like Goliath, it is a giant with a fatal weakness. When the public is educated about its techniques, it often loses its ability to mislead and manipulate".

According to the egalitarian voice, public relations operates by stealth, because it proposes tradeoffs relating to the value of human life that it cannot defend in public. The egalitarian voice searches for a treacherous tradeoff to publicise and thereby mobilise outrage. This provides riveting entertainment for the mass media and gives public relations's dominant coalition indigestion. Stauber and Rampton this tack in pointing to the inherent corruption of corporate public relations. "The need to maximise profit drove antifreeze makers to hire a PR spy so they could fight a lawthatwould save children's lives at a price of only two cents a gallon".

Unmasking public relations's deceits is difficult because public relations practitioners conceal their work. Rampton and Stauber took aim at public relations's cultivated use of third party expert endorsements. The guiding mantra for public relations practitioners was to "put your words in someone else's mouth. The 'someone elses' become Potemkin authorities, faithfully spouting the opinions of their benefactors while making it appear that their views are 'independent'". This approach "offers camouflage, helping to hide the vested interests that lurks behind a message".

Public relations's egalitarian critics are particularly critical of "pseudograssroots" movements. "Astroturf" organising deprives social movements of their natural advantage in public debates: public skepticism about the intentions of corporate interests. "Recognising that industry lacks credibility on environmental issues, industry's public relations modus operandi often is to create front groups to advocate its interests sometimes well-cloaked, other times thinly veiled, and always with Orwellian names". Front groups enable "corporations to take part in public debates and government hearings behind a cover of community concern". "Astroturf public relations" confuses the public as to who the heroes and the villains are. This sows doubt about the authenticity of the egalitarian voice and makes it difficult to mobilise outrage.

In recent years, the egalitarian voice has begun to articulate an affirmative vision of public relations that embraces a communitarian ethic. Public relations scholars have been at the head of this effort. The affirmative egalitarian vision proposes to reform corporate public relations along egalitarian lines and to expand the definition of public relations to include the organising activities of activist groups. The reformers propose to rebuild public relations on the usable parts of public relations practice.

"Community relations is the paradigm case of public relations". Public relations should embrace community building. Interest in community welfare, social order, and progress can be addressed by public relations practitioners. As a social center, through a concern for art and a concern for community play, the organisation can help to enhance community. Practitioners can help the community share aesthetic experience, religious ideas, personal values, and sentiments. Practitioners will not only do advocacy, but also will foster communication that "offers an immediate enhancement of life, which can be enjoyed for its own sake". The feminist critique of public relations is the most developed egalitarian effort to transform corporate public relations.

Feminist research has identified structural changes that are necessary to make public relations a more equitable profession, including making public relations's body of knowledge more inclusive and gender sensitive. These inquiries have sensitised researchers to the inequitable power arrangements in gendered relationships and have increased the discipline's sensitivity to the experiences of public relations practitioners. Although some practitioners have worried that the increasing proportion of female practitioners threatens the organisational status of public relations, feminist theorists believe that "women's emergence in public relations is an opportunity for a more responsible and effective practice".

The discipline will be transformed as students and practitioners come to embrace feminist values (e.g., cooperation, valuing relationships, altruism). The classroom may be the ideal setting in which to consider that the development of personal feminist values that have implications for public relations practice. Such consideration would benefit all students and may be an important step toward realisation of our aspirations for a practice that is truly professional, truly ethical and truly effective. Explicitly embracing feminist values should "help define the field and, in particular, clarify its purposes. Those purposes such as reinstitution of community, the development of relationships, and the resolution of conflict will be grounded in the character of those who work in public relations".

Egalitarian theorists insist that public relations must embrace diversity for both moral and practical reasons. As every domain of public relations practice becomes more diverse, "practitioners and educators must become more sensitive to this environmental change by enacting diversity as a concern relevant to their professional lives and by responding to it interactively". Instead of seeking similarity and harmony, we need to recruit people and pursue ideas that challenge the status quo.We should not just seek out identifiable minorities, but also people who have demonstrated a sensitivity to cultural diversity and a commitment to helping others become responsive to it.

The affirmative egalitarian vision of public relations also seeks to expand the definition of public relations. The activities of activist groups are also within the boundaries of public relations. Smith argued, "The exclusion, or misrepresentation, of activist organisations in the scholarly and pedagogical literature limits our understanding of public relations". The distinction between organisational public relations and social movements is a false dichotomy. Activists must organise to pursue their goals. Once they do, they also "face challenges that require public relations programmes". The activist organisation must compete with other activist organisations for attention and resources to maintain its membership. "One of the realities of activism is that simple survival requires a great deal of time and energy".

Critical theorists criticise public relations research because it subsidises "commercial and state communications at the expense of other segments of the population". Public relations research has "privileged or subsidised certain segments of the population and marginalised others to the periphery of public discourse". Public relations's body of knowledge is inaccessible to most people. Only commercial and state entities have the professional experience and material resources to apply the body of knowledge. Public relations scholars should develop knowledge that equips ordinary citizens to enter into public discourse. "Public communication skills and resources must be extended to all segments of society if communication symmetry is to be recognised". Researchers should focus on the "types of communication practices that are within the reach of resource poor segments of society".

Public relations can contribute to grassroots democracy through activism and radical politics. Pointing to the inevitable contradictions within public relations's ideology, "This perspective opens the door for public relations practitioners to act as community activists, an approach that is not only radical but also ethical and desirable". Enlarging the scope of public relations will require dramatic shifts in public relations education. "The field's case studies, texts and research give preference to public relations as a management function of capitalist organisations, including state organisations". This will involve some conflict among practitioners, as "public relations practitioners line up on opposite sides of the trenches, but so do legal practitioners, marketing experts, and many other professionals in everyday life".

The postmodern environment will be so turbulent that the predictive tools of social science will be of little use. "Hot issue publics and the media skills of activists call into question the ability to deal proactively with activists". Fluid interactions between organisations and publics will replace issues management. For the postmodern version of public relations, it will "be the responsibility of the public relations function to create opportunities for dissent, for opening up debate without forcing consensus, to create possibilities for change".

Tactics are not the product of careful cold reason, they do not follow a table of organisation or plan of attack. Accident, unpredictable reactions to your actions, necessity and improvisation dictate the direction and nature of tactics...the tactic itself comes out of the free flow of action and reaction. The egalitarian voice differentiates between strategic public relations and public relations tactics. It is anxious that the strategic use of public relations by large organisations subverts participatory democracy, but the egalitarian voice embraces public relations tactics as essential tools for promoting social change.

In the parallel egalitarian movement of public journalism, publicity emerged as an essential tool for mobilising action and developing community. Rejecting "strategy" and embracing "tactics" is faithful to the underlying egalitarian tendency to value spontaneity in action. Although it is often excluded from the debates of public relations's dominant coalition, the egalitarian voice has profoundly influenced public relations practice. It makes the cultures of the dominant coalition nervous. As a gadfly culture, the egalitarian voice is always ready to sting. In its affirmative form, it seeks to make public relations work for the common good. It is not yet a part of public relations's dominant coalition, but its influence is increasing.

Hierarchical Voice

The hierarchical voice has long been a member of public relations's dominant coalition, along with the CI voice. It frequently appears in accounts of public relations history and practice. It aims to improve the status of public relations and to institutionalise public relations as a core management function. It has used public relations history to enhance the discipline's status. Its version of public relations history depicts a process of steady evolutionary progress. Despite its origins in the tawdry practice of press agentry, public relations has come of age as a knowledge based discipline.

Edward Bernays consistently articulated the hierarchical voice. Bernays portrayed public relations counselors as societal psychotherapists. "Society has become more complex and its processes have been speeded up over the last few centuries. The rate of progress of the many forces that make up society has been uneven with consequently increased maladjustment and tension". Bernays wanted to solve irrational communication problems. "Maladjustments in many fields, commerce, industry, religion, and government, are based upon the misunderstanding of realities and communications processes....Conflict that is based on misunderstanding, ignorance, and apathy is unnecessary and wasteful".

Bernays saw public relations as "a vital tool of adjustment, interpretation, and integration between individuals, groups and society". Public relations "is vitally important today because modern social science has found that the adjustment of individuals, groups, and institutions to life is necessary for the well-being of all". It is an activity "that makes competition, another factor of our society, more efficient and effective". The public relations counselor must overcome the ignorance of clients and publics. Although the "highest level of adjustment is reached at the point of enlightened self-interest. The public relations counsel must ensure that such enlightenment prevails [italics added]". Bernays recognised that much of public relations practice fell short of the hierarchical ideal. He attributed this imperfection to the lack of controlled barriers to entry into the profession.

"There are too few trained and skilled practitioners. In the early years of the profession, many crowded in who had little specialised knowledge, aptitude or experience". Throughout his life, Bernays championed the cause of licensing public relations practitioners. He thought licensing would help secure public relations's boundaries and exclude unscrupulous and incompetent practitioners. Bernays remained optimistic about public relations's prospects and projected a rising curve of disciplinary growth and maturation. Life in the democratic age was vexing, but with advice of public relations counselors, leaders could navigate these rapids with confidence.

The hierarchical preference for dispassionate expertise also appeared in Hill's account of how Hill and Knowlton operated. Hill was proud that his firm was the first to

a) Offer a broad range of specialised public relations services.

b) Apply cost accounting and budgeting procedures to agency work.

c) Develop an international presence in public relations.

d) Create a professional research division.

He celebrated the breadth and depth of his professional staff by reciting their years of public relations experience, their educational pedigrees, and their international experiences. Displaying a faith in the hierarchical themes of content specialisation and hierarchical integration, he wrote, "Only by such a variegated grouping of education, experience, talent and linguistic capabilities can a large public relations firm meet the requirements of its clients".

Hill portrayed public relations work as a dignified enterprise. He believed that teamwork among experts would "replace the lone-wolf operator-the 'Big I Ams'-as an important factor in the public relations business". He insisted that his firm not solicit business because "we have tried over a period of three and a half decades to build a reputation for high standards of service". Referrals from existing clients provided the needed business. In a tone similar to current manifestos of relationship marketing, Hill opined, "The relations of public relations firms with their clients ordinarily is intimate and deeply immersed in policies and activities". He wrote, "Fortunately, the public relations counseling business is unlike advertising in that among the top grade firms the shifting of accounts from one firm to another is indeed a rarity".

Philip Lesly represented a more pessimistic strain of the hierarchical viewpoint. Surveying the rise of egalitarian movements in the United States, Lesly counseled executives on how to prevail over the forces of anarchy. Lesly was pessimistic about the possibilities for societal adjustment and integration. He believed that egalitarianism was a rising menace that needed to be neutralised.

Lesly asserted "The first responsibility of an executive is to create and maintain orderly procedures....The effective manager is naturally repelled by disorder and threats to smooth operations". The climate of public opinion was "an attack upon leadership. It presumes that all organisations are suspect and that the leaders of those organisations are probably scoundrels or oppressors". He feared that hierarchy would be "replaced by a tyranny of the crowd, in which the assertiveness of groups of people prevents any orderly functioning". Executives must defend their organisations. "It is evident on all sides that it is those who defy authority disclaim any responsibility for their in-surgence; and it is the established institution that needs to defend itself against siege".

Lesly also lamented the "balkanisation" of public relations. Public relations was increasing in its scope, but itspoweris being dissipatedbycompetition for the spotlightamongitsvaried practitioners. Each function of the field...is seeking to define itself as public relations, rather than recognising that it is onlyoneelementin averybroadfield. In defining the field, one should "stress the gestalt of public relations rather than the segment. Give primacy to the really vital functions and base everything in public relations education to breadth and depth".

Lesly preferred a far-sighted systems-oriented perspective. The hierarchical voice for public relations shares the common desires for (a) distinct boundaries for defining public relations, (b) a definitive body of knowledge that hierarchy can apply, and (c) regulative mechanisms to defend the boundaries of public relations (i.e., keep charlatans and unqualified persons out of the profession). The stock arguments of the hierarchical voice have been quite consistent. If an applied social science approach is taken, public relations can develop a body of theoretic knowledge that meets and distinguishes the practice of public relations from the craft of the communication technician....Such a body of knowledge...is the foundation stone on which public relations can develop more and more professionalism. A standardised body of knowledge would guide public relations practice, help standardise public relations curricula, generate respect for the profession, and repel the epitaphs of "public relations flack."

A body of knowledge would ease hierarchy's fears about the discipline's foundations. Many believe that public relations theory and scholarship are steadily progressing toward this goal. The aim is to integrate relevant knowledge into a systemic and predictive theory. For instance, crisis public relations is moving from crisis communication toward anticipatory models of crisis management. Where media planning once required little planning, the current situation is starkly different. The sheer number of publicity outlets has expanded, increasing the direct costs to provide materials and making it difficult to approach every potential outlet effectively.

In this more complex media landscape, public relations practitioners need to "practice and think about media broadly and strategically. An effective public relations programme must employ techniques ranging from broad-based traditional mass communication to highly individualised interpersonal communication. Moreover, the process of selecting media must be rationalised". However, some fear that the process of "rationalisation" is not proceeding fast enough. Speaking of the "fad" of integrated marketing communication (IMC), "is little more than a confession that nonintegrated or disintegrated communications have been the norm in the past".

The real debate should be about the "relationship between what might be termed integrated marketing and integrated communication". However, this debate was not being engaged because public relations was unilaterally ceding its turf to marketing, as "marketing scholars and practitioners are methodically redefining marketing as public relations". Some of the organisational functions were assimilating high-order public relations functions such as investor relations. This was not due to marketing imperialism, so much as it was due to the failure of public relations scholarship to "define itself and to develop sophisticated and progressive theory".

In the view of some practitiners the legitimacy of the public relations function was precarious. "There remains a need for public relations to define its intellectual and practical domain, especially vis-á-vis marketing, to regain control over its destiny". Within the hierarchical tribe, the optimists and pessimists disagree on the soundness of the discipline's intellectual underpinnings. The ambitious projects of the hierarchical voice are far from completion. The hierarchical voice faces formidable cultural challenges. In particular, the CI voice objects that public relations practice is too situational, fluid, and emergent to be thoroughly rationalised. Despite these challenges, many hierarchical adherents remain optimistic, anticipating that the 21st century will be the golden age of public relations.

AI Voice

AI is the refuge of the free spirit. "This way of life is distinguished from the other four 'engaged' ways of life by its intellectual independence and lofty detachment". For enlightenment to be attained, human nature must be liberated from attachment and dependency. AIs avoid coercive entanglements, especially coercive demands for "right thinking." Human relationships must have exit points; individuals must be able to withdraw from associations that become oppressive. "To the extent that we are capable of detaching ourselves from the fray and rising above it, we are likely to appreciate the partiality of those below".

Cultural theory considers the AI culture to be rare. However, Fiske's equality matching model showed how AI interdependence is structured. An equality matching relationship maintains equality of input and reward (e.g., two couples trade babysitting services). In work settings, equality matching synchronises the contributions of group members so that each works at the same rate. Equality matching ensures that neither party accumulates long term debt. This exchange minimises long term dependence and maintains mutual autonomy. To the extent that the AI culture participates in public relations discussions, it mainly seeks to preserve a public relations niche for cooperative and noncoercive relationships.

In politics, the Natural Law Party articulates the AI voice. Human problems "result from a narrowness of vision that fails to comprehend life's essential unity". However, "with maximally expanded comprehension, individuals naturally behave in their own best long term interests while promoting the interests of society as a whole action fully aligned with natural law". With proper enlightenment, the need for governmental regulation will diminish. People who practice public relations as a part time craft may represent this position. Some public relations partnerships have features similar to the AI model.

In a study of executive conflict, found a work culture that characterised as "silent hives." The social relationships in these partnership firms maximised professional autonomy, discretion, and equality. They

also minimised overt expressions of conflict. In agency public relations, partners may share the costs of doing business, while each practitioner maintains his or her own accounts and independent areas of expertise.

If information is a "neutral medium," one can function as a journalist in residence by responding to inquiries about the organisation. In a more proactive form, one might put out information for people to use as they see fit. An AI representative might prefer the job title of "information specialist." The AI perspective provides scholars with an important refuge. The "intellectual domain requires a conscious uncoupling of intellectual agenda from the thoughts, actions and preoccupations of practitioners". For most people, the AI perspective represents a temporary stopping point.

"Adherents to the different engaged ways of life argue with each other with different premises, but often reserve a special contempt for philosophers who merely interpret". The AI framework encourages one to stand aloof from social life. Adams speculated that AI might "induce a resigned fatalism or provide the three activist ways of life with superior insight into the behavior of competing ideologies, an insight that they may seek to exploit in their own management of risk". Practitioners must have a "breadth of perspective" to interpret management to publics and vice versa. However, public relations practitioners had such a comprehensive perspective. A practitioner's organisational position and role limits her vision. "Theoretically, it is questionable that practitioners can develop the perspective they have claimed to offer".

However, the AI perspective does not require superhuman intuition because the relational models are part of our social knowledge. Perspective taking requires a clear memory to avoid cultural myopia.

CI Voice

The CI voice is a powerful voice in the dominant public relations coalition. The CI voice celebrates public relations practice as a virtuoso performance. CI culture cultivates the biography of the great person. Ivy Lee articulated this voice in the discipline's infancy. Hiebert's historical biography of Leecaptured the CIspirit. Hiebert wrote, "Lee was impressed by the important and newsworthy people. He made the most to cultivate his contacts with prominent men and then in making an impression with his own talents and personality".

According to Hiebert, "Lee's respect for the great men of his time never waned". Lee chastised his associate Daniel Pierce by saying, "Dan, you spend toomuchtime with unimportant people". Leeassiduously cultivated this network of influential people. Hiebert concluded that Lee "put himself squarely into the circle of his day. From his position hewas able to win wide respect for the new profession of public relations". Lee held his ground with the titans of industry as he promoted his mantra of informing the public. Hiebert noted that Lee was "one of the few men who could make millionaires wait for him". Lee was a 20th century Renaissance Man. He had more than 10,000 books in his library and could quote verbatim from many hundreds of them.

Hiebert wrote that Lee was most interested in "the spread of ideas in which he believed. Indeed his disregard for money bordered on improvidence". Lee had an eclectic interest "in the whole range of human relationships, trade, employee, industrial, government, community and international". In contrast to the specialised tasks of Hill's public relations, Lee sought intuitive solutions. Bernays characterised Lee's work as an "art" and labeled his own work as more "scientific". In an era of knowledge explosion, expertise becomes

increasingly narrow and hinders decision making. Brummet argued that disciplines like public relations must use narrative to reduce the complexity of public domain communications to manageable proportions. The CI voice bristles at the hierarchical strictures of corporate public relations.

In another venue, complained that bureaucratic corporate cultures were subverting public relations practice. "Public relations managers themselves are quarantined from the daily combat of opinion making by staff and staff is cushioned from accountability by specialisation". Public relations is "a unique profession. Because it deals with the unpredictable-opinions, attitudes, impressions-it has to be flexible, dynamic, instantaneous and exceptionally skilled". The dynamic environment of public relations meant that public relations "must be entrepreneurial not bureaucratic! In attitudes, approach and activity".

The CI voice emphasises the contextual variations of public relations. Public relations theory cannot encompass all of the unique niches that public relations contains. Moreover, the public relations environment is always changing. Theory lags behind practice and is often outmoded by the time it is developed. New professionals must have apprenticeships and practical experience to learn the ropes.

You simply cannot learn public relations from a book. This belief in flux and change appears in how the CI voice constructs the public relations implications of the Internet. Where the hierarchical voice projects that the Internet will be integrated with existing public relations practices, the CI voice declares that public relations needs to be reinvented to fit the world of the Internet. The Internet offers just another message delivery tool, with limited and impatient audiences. This view is on par with the horse-and-buggy operator criticising the Model-T

Ford for being too loud. The Internet is not just a new medium; it's rapidly becoming a platform for all other media, and more. In the end, the CI voice is not anxious about names or labels.

Ivy Lee never selected one label to describe what he did, "confessing at the end of his life that even his own children did not know what to call him". The CI voice is more concerned with making things happen than it is with definitions and labels. CI culture exudes confidence about the future. It will be the best of times for those who are willing to learn and willing to grasp the rings of power.

IMPLICATIONS FOR PUBLIC RELATIONS

CT framework also applies to discourse about public relations. Of course, many debates within public relations do not organise themselves around the CT presented here. Many debates concern issues where scholars and practitioners share the same CT. Such debates often focus on the best means to accomplish agreed on ends or about the adequacy of current attempts to build the discipline's knowledge base. These debates may seldom articulate their underlying cultural premises. It is also true that a person may shift in her cultural allegiances over time.

It is also true that the same person may express different CT at the same point in time, especially if the speaker crosses domains. Adams reminded us that "Our cultural filters must cope with a cacophony of competing and conflicting messages. ... But often it appears that our lives are compartmentalised in ways that permit us to hold beliefs that are mutually inconsistent". However, even this seeming inconsistency may be reconciled if one admits that different models of relationships apply to different parts of the social world. Shifts in CT across time and domains do not undermine the CT framework.

Indeed, the CT system can make these transitions intelligible.

The CT system identifies the limited number of rhetorical options that a speaker has for arguing for the correctness of social practices. The CT perspective identifies likely points of opposition and engagement between the different cultural camps. The twists and turns of cultural discourse can be complex, but a CT perspective allows one to anticipate and interpret these constructions. Futurework will determine howuseful theCT framework is for interpreting specific issues within public relations. Several projects areworthy of mention. The CT framework could identify cases of "toxic public relations discourse."

Historical critique of the dark side of egalitarian political discourse is an exemplar of howsuchwork could proceed. Rhetorical critiques could identify "cultural pathologies" that emerge when a particular cultural voice becomes hegemonic. Future research should also investigate how each cultural tribe constructs public relations's history. This could include an analysis of how each cultural camp constructs its cultural adversaries to advance its own proposals for the discipline. Such analyses also could chart how public relations discourse has shifted from one set of cultural pre-suppositions to another. For instance, a "cultural history" of how the two-way symmetrical model of public relations has evolved is certainly in order. Also need to determine what kinds of cultural diversity enhance public relations practice. In addition to ethnic diversity, cultural theory asserts that cultural diversity is a necessity for democratic life.

3

PURCHASING PUBLIC RELATIONS

Good public relations raises share-prices, catapults products into brand-leadership and turns enemies into allies. Incompetent public relations destroys products, careers and investor support overnight. Securing the very best public relations services must be high on any organisation's agenda. The public relations consultancy sector in the UK is world-class but surprisingly small. Professional procurement executives are increasingly involved in selecting public relations consultancies and managing their terms of engagement.

Public relations practitioners operate across a wider range than any other business or professional service from briefing a Government Minister to writing a press release to negotiating with a Non-Governmental Organisation -and this can make it hard to determine exactly what they do, what they can be expected to do, and what they should be paid. The Public Relations Consultants Association (PRCA) has produced to help clarify some of these questions. The first part tries to explain what public relations consultancy is and does; the second part concentrates on the more technical aspects of selecting consultancies and negotiating contracts.

Greater involvement and support on the part of procurement professionals will add rigour to the process of selecting public relations consultancies, setting their terms of reference, negotiating their remuneration and monitoring their performance. It will help to focus effort on desired business outcomes rather than just PR activities. In this way we will be able to work together to make tangible the value delivered by PR consultancy.

ROLE OF PUBLIC RELATIONS CONSULTANCIES

Public relations works exceptionally well in UK, which has led to rapid growth and a high degree of specialisation. There are now 200 substantial public relations consultancies in this country—many managing global or European programmes on behalf of UK clients—and 2,000 small partnerships or individual practitioners. The services they provide to client organisations are diverse.

Financial communications and investor relations: corporate communications, which may include Corporate Social Responsibility, issues & crisis management and liaison with stakeholder groups; public affairs at local, national and EU level; product support, including retailer relations, launches and promotions; sponsorship in arts, sports and the community; internal communications and change management... Most consultancies have a strong core competence in media relations—preparing editorial material for broadcast, web and print outlets and managing relationships between clients and their key media; and nearly all are expert at event management - staging meetings, writing speeches and presentations and maximising the impact of a corporate event or a client's participation in a public occasion.

The common factor in this varied landscape is skill in communication. A good public relations consultancy will be able to master a brief rapidly, design a communication programme to achieve the stated business result, create original materials to attract attention and change opinion, and report on the degree of change which has been achieved. The business model of most public relations consultancies resembles that of a legal or accountancy practice. The role of management is to balance client demand—usually expressed in hours or days per assignment per senior/junior specialist/generalist consultant—against available resources. Most consultancies invest in talent ahead of known demand. Consultancies' overheads are largely fixed and are allocated over the coming fiscal year on a straight-line basis.

A percentage of every consultant's hour or day charged is therefore accounted for by rent, IT systems and office support costs. Management exercise discretion in the level of investment they make in knowledge acquisition and maintenance and in training and professional development. Most consultancies seek to improve margins by offering services which are visibly better, often in specialist areas, and therefore able to command a premium in the marketplace. Awards, publications, research and the hiring of "star recruits" all contribute to the looked-for differentiation between a consultancy and its competitors. A strong track-record in a particular field, a name for exceptional creativity, or possession of a good international network, are also clearly apparent methods of establishing points of difference.

The majority of consultancies' account teams are made up of an account director, who will be the focal point of the relationship with the client, and one or more account managers and account executives. A board director, usually with a named deputy, will provide overall guidance, advice and knowledge based on their greater experience. In many cases specialists—in, for example, political or internal communications—will be assigned to the team on a temporary or part-time basis.

VALUE OF PUBLIC RELATIONS CONSULTANCY

The importance of maintaining a good corporate reputation, and the desirability of securing more than a fair share of attention in the marketing arena, are generally accepted by most organisations in the UK today. This is good evidence for the effectiveness of the practice of public relations. Yet three questions continually confront clients:

- How much of our public relations work should be undertaken in-house, and how much is best outsourced?
- How can we determine the optimum amount to invest in public relations?
- How can we reliably assess the relative value offered by consultancies, both before an engagement begins and at review?

The answer to the first question varies according to the size and complexity of the client organisation and according to the inclination of the in-house communications director or public relations chief. Most consultancies will have advice to offer on all three questions, and this is one of their most valuable contributions at the strategic level. Consultancies can help in four principal ways:

- A good consultancy can offer exceptionally expert people, usually with a diverse range of experience, who can complement the knowledge and ideas of the in-house public relations team.
- Consultancies will usually be able to bring experience from other industries and possibly other countries to bear on the issue at hand, thus

exposing the in-house team to ideas cross-fertilised from completely different business areas.

— Consultancies are designed elastically, so are ready and able to provide many-handed support, at a moment's notice, in times of emergency or peak demand.

— Because they exist outside the corporate structure, consultants can offer observations and advice which are objective and impartial.

Calculating the right amount to invest in public relations is extremely difficult. Companies in the same industry sector can be seen allocating widely differing budgets to public relations, sometimes in the order of 500 per cent. Much depends on whether the client organisation sees itself as a "challenger", in which case—typically—higher-than average investments in profile and marketing will pay back as market-share increases, or as a "defender" of an existing market position, in which case expenditure may be minimised in order to favour margin.

In most instances, the client organisation will have an existing involvement in public relations. So there will be benchmarks against which to review budget adjustments. Clients frequently invite the consultancy market to help determine the optimum budget by soliciting tenders based solely on (a) a commercial objective, or (b) a tightly-defined scope of work, sometimes expressed as a set of deliverables or as a specific improvement across a range of existing benchmarks. When a client wishes to take a completely fresh look at public relations investment, it is usually in tandem with marketing and communications expenditure across the board. A number of analytical tools exist to help allocate budgets between the various communications channels.

Procurement professionals can help their colleagues achieve value by ensuring that every assignment has a framework of deliverables, milestones, key performance indicators and essential measures of success, and that the consultancy commits to this framework as the core of its proposal. Comparing relative value offered by public relations consultancies at the outset of an engagement, or at a competitive review, is necessarily a combination of objective and subjective judgements. Research shows that experience, creativity and chemistry are normally the three key factors in consultancy selection. Value for money is generally recognised as being difficult to gauge. Yet this is, perhaps, the key focus of procurement professionals. The PRCA recommends a series of questions which may help to determine comparative value in a consultancy review:

— Recent and relevant experience in the client's industry sector and/or in a communications programme similar to the brief.

— The presence on the engagement team of individual practitioners with relevant experience and demonstrable insight into the communications challenges and solutions.

— Capacity to devote sufficient time and expertise to the assignment without over-stretching resources. For example: how many clients, and what size of programmes, does each team-member handle?

— Ability to bring specialist communications skills to bear on the problems: for example, experts in NGO liaison, sponsorship, webcasting, product placement, guerrilla marketing, internal communications, community relations as appropriate.

— A track-record of long-established and successful relationships with organisations of your type and culture.

— Demonstration of better-than-average staff retention, and evidence of serious commitment to training and career development.

— Cost-effective proposals for measuring the success of the programme—either in its entirety or via selected key elements which can be isolated and evaluated. Most consultancies use measurement tools authenticated by the PRCA and IPR, or have developed proprietary systems, or recommend the involvement of an independent evaluation specialist.

— Overall... an understanding on the part of all team members of the contribution which public relations can make to the business objectives of the organisation.

For over thirty years in the UK the public relations industry has made a consistent effort to determine and publish professional standards of behaviour, performance and accountability. There are two principal bodies involved in this pursuit: The Public Relations Consultants Association (PRCA), whose focus is consulting firms, and the Institute of Public Relations (IPR), whose members are individuals working in-house, in consultancies or in the academic world as teachers or students. Members of the PRCA have all obtained the Consultancy Management Standard, independently audited by Det Norske Veritas (DNV). They must also abide by the PRCA's Professional Charter and Codes of Conduct. Members of the IPR must satisfy a range of criteria to join and progress from "associate" to "member" to "fellow".

Some consultancies have earned investors in people accreditation, ISO certification or other independent marks of professional and commercial competence. Specialist consultancies in public affairs or healthcare, for example, may belong to the Association of Professional Political Consultants (APPC) or the Healthcare Communications Association (HCA), while financial and investor relations specialists may belong to the Investor Relations Society (IRS). Many large client organisations now require that rostered public relations consultancies must demonstrate appropriate certification, in particular the PRCA's Consultancy Management Standard.

Most public relations consultancies base their charges on the hourly rate of the individuals comprising the client's account team, multiplied by the number of hours each person devotes to the client's programme. These hourly rates tend to be similar between consultancies for the same kind of consultant (experience, track-record, degree of specialist knowledge). The value and cost differential between one consultancy and another lies in the quality of the practitioners they employ and the quality of the support—knowledge, research, IT systems, training, career development, leadership, management—they deploy. Public relations consultancy contracts are normally of four types:

— A set fee for a specific project with a beginning, middle and end.

— A taximeter system for engagements where the level of service is likely to vary widely— including no requirement at all from time to time.

— An annual retainer based on a pre-determined work requirement and a set schedule of deliverables.

— A retainer with an agreement for over-hours to be charged when unexpected demand occurs.

Many public relations assignments start on a project basis and evolve into retainer-plus-over-hours once trust and an appreciation of good value have developed. Most consultancies will charge a standard price for work carried out during the normal working week but a premium price for services provided after-hours, at weekends and during public holidays, or in emergencies. Costs in other countries vary considerably, from 200 per cent of the UK average to 25 per cent in developing markets. Expenses and office costs may be charged item-by-item, or may be charged as an all-in percentage of the budget, or may be absorbed within the overall service fee.

Purchases (photography, print, events and so on) may be charged to the client after consultancy sign-off, or may be paid and re-billed by the consultancy with an agreed additional handling charge. Many consultancies propose an element of payment-by-results within their overall compensation. This is often the case in financial communications, where success fees are a frequent component of inter-firm agreements, and also in engagements where the looked-for result is solely attributable to the consultancy. The PRCA and the ISBA have developed a standard contract, which is available from either organisation.

NEGOTIATING WITH PUBLIC RELATIONS PEOPLE

Public relations consultancy managers may be entrepreneurs, but that they are first and-foremost public relations practitioners. Only at the largest firms will you encounter trained negotiators or professional counterparts to yourselves. The PRCA offers the following signposts in the hope that they will help conclude a mutually successful agreement:

— Ascertain and compare the hourly/daily rates charged by each consultancy for each "rank" of practitioner. Determine how each firm defines its "ranks"—executives, managers, account directors and so on —so as to be sure that you are comparing like with like. Similarly, how will the team be put together? Will the consultancy need to recruit additional people? For a large programme this is inevitable.

— Enquire how each consultancy handles purchases made on your behalf. Is a handling-charge levied?

If not, and suppliers' bills are submitted to you directly, does the consultancy take responsibility for checking quality, cost and timely supply?

— How will the consultancies invest in the success of the relationship? For example: will they absorb all or some of the costs of the learning curve? Will their most senior people be available to advise? Most public relations firms are hoping for long-term engagements with new clients: how will the contenders for your account go about building a partnership with your organisation?

— What Key Performance Indicators and what core deliverables do the consultancies envisage as being crucial to the success of the programme? How do the consultancies propose to monitor client team satisfaction -how often, and by what methods?

— Do you see the assignment as routine, important or business-critical?

— Is it clear to the consultancies how you will make your selection?

— Which methods of measurement and evaluation do the consultancies believe are most suitable to the assignment? Have you set aside a separate budget for this function?

— Are the consultancies ready to negotiate a proportion of their compensation on a payment-by-results basis? Are you prepared to offer a bonus for exceptional performance? The PRCA's Consultancy Management Standard The PRCA's Consultancy Management Standard was the world's first independently-audited quality certification scheme for public relations consultancies. Introduced in the UK in 2000 after three years of development, it is being adopted in ten other countries and is the model for similar schemes throughout the world.

The Standard was designed to give clients the assurance that a certified consultancy is financially stable, well-managed, adheres to best practice in all dimensions of client service, invests in training its staff, has a convincing strategy for the development of its business, abides by the principles of the PRCA's professional charter, and adheres to the PRCA's Codes of Conduct. Member consultancies are re-examined every two years by DNV.

4

PUBLIC RELATION AND THE MOTIVE

Public relations helps an organisation and its publics adapt mutually to each other. Business schools teach profit maximisation, transferring wealth from customers to owners, because that is what business does. Commerce is unlike medicine where lifesaving is at the core of what doctors do, or engineering where improving mankind's lot is at the heart of calculations. Commerce is about exchange of goods, services and wealth. There needn't be any ethic other than completion of a transaction. One can complete business transactions with illegal and injurious products and services as well as with offerings that are for the betterment of mankind. It is up to company leadership and to societal regulators to make sure companies remain within the boundaries of accepted societal ethics. On the other hand, PR teaches relationship and reputation building in ways that lead to profits.

PR assumes a business has vested interested in ethics. We know, of course, that this isn't true. And, concerns for reputation and relationships can be addressed as easily in illegitimate businesses as in legitimate ones. A madam can run a whorehouse with an eye to treating customers well, so they return often, and a drug dealer can protect product from harmful contamination that might kill users and diminish cash flow. As PR practitioners, we advocate reputation and relationships to company leadership that sometimes listens and sometimes doesn't. We point to societal pressure, often expressed through governmental action and news stories, that can revoke a company's permission to operate if it steps too far over the line of what society deems acceptable behavior. But a direct link to revenues and profits is missing unless a company is in a disaster scenario. There is even more conflict.

Under financial assumptions, money now is more important than money later. Reaping the greatest wealth today from customers for shareholders is better than doing so tomorrow. Under PR principles, money later is as valuable as money now, if one wants an enterprise to which customers return repeatedly and stand by loyally. In a business school view, one maintains reputation and relationships to produce revenues and earnings.

For public relations, reputation and relationships lead to revenue and profits. The points of view appear identical, but practically speaking they aren't because business people, like business school professors, forget part of the equation. Business school professors tend to abstract profit from the business context, while public relations holds that the business context is essential-profit comes from flesh-and-blood people engaging in transactions. Put another way, in business schools, there appears to be more emphasis on mathematics than on messy details of customer, vendor and employee relationships and reputations.

FINANCE TYRANNY

In fairness to business schools, many offer real-world experiences to students in to give them a better feel for the totality of business. But too often real-world courses are optional and attendant lessons in leadership, communications and ethics are good things to do but not essential. Communications or public relations courses in business schools are not mainstream, and perhaps never will be.

Finance professors are often first among equals and financial theory and calculation are considered more important than organisational theory and psychology. Students manipulate numbers without reference to people who turn numbers into facts. Too often, financially trained MBAs become quantitatively oriented consultants unskilled in leadership, communications and ethics necessary for making products, completing sales and serving customers for the long term.

Few ever run stores or factories, even though these can be large enterprises. A big-box, do-it-yourself store can produce Rs. 50 crore in annual sales with all the problems attendant to retailing including staffing, logistics, shrink, training, communications and customer service. But, it is not uncommon that managers running these stores and responsible for a business' primary relationships are not college graduates. Relationship and reputation management are at the core of marketing but even so, academic discussion often turns on abstract considerations and mathematical models rather than practical considerations of how to handle a customer who has just purchased Rs. 900,000 of kitchen cabinetry and finds it doesn't fit.

However, what business schools teach is responsive to their market-large corporations, consulting firms and Wall Street financial houses that hire business school graduates. A gauge of a business school's success is the number of graduates employed by prestigious companies at high starting salaries. These businesses want the analytical skills of MBAs and reward them proportionately. It may be that businesses hiring MBAs do not understand the need for reputation and relationships (which is unlikely), or they assume business students, as well as business persons, come equipped with ethical skills. But the problem turns quickly into one of focus, especially on Wall Street.

Pursuit of wealth is at the heart of investors' participation in markets. They prefer money now, although they can be suckers for a story that profits will come later - as happened during the Internet Bubble. Capital is impatient and institutional investors demand return. They are not shareholder loyalists, if a company fails to perform, and they rarely focus on the totality of a business or consider reputation and relationships when reviewing portfolios. Investors are angry when scandal and fraud diminish the value of investments, but they are not necessarily upset by how a company relates to other target audiences, such as employees, customers and vendors, even if there are violations of human rights.

Governments pass laws, such as the Sarbanes-Oxley Law of 2002, to forbid practices that penalise shareholders and institute reforms that reduce the possibility of fraud. These reforms barely extend beyond investors to employees and others who are part of a universe of reputation and relationships that comprise a business. Other laws apply to them, but investors may not take such laws into account except in how they affect a company's revenue and earnings potential. Sharp focus on the bottom-line assumes, or forgets, too much. Companies in highly competitive environments with driven CEOs tend to forget the wider context of ethics, reputation and relationships in pursuit of revenues and earnings that "keep the Street happy." Business schools teaching profit maximisation also tend to forget that numbers are not isolated abstractions.

There is an irony that a foremost proponent of reputation and relationship principles was the senior PR person at a monopoly - AT&T --, which wasn't subject to real-world competition when Arthur W. Page developed public relations philosophy and principles. And as a consequence of his actions and example, as well as his many speeches, letters, and presentations, he fashioned a model of public relations and public relations performance that today remains the ideal to which all of us aspire. American Telephone & Telegraph. Page's philosophy centered about understanding and communicating corporate and individual character. He emphasised humanism and freedom as preconditions for capitalism. He stressed that a "successful corporation must shape its character in concert with the nation's. It must operate in the public interest, manage for the long run and make customer satisfaction its primary goal".

"Real success, both for big business and the public, lies in large enterprise conducting itself in the public interest and in such a way that the public will give it sufficient freedom to serve effectively." Open most finance and accounting books, and you won't find that view expressed. A company in a benign monopoly is concerned about keeping captive customers happy and not just keeping customers. And indeed, when AT&T lost its monopoly, it faded to a shadow. Companies fighting in tough marketplaces prefer sales-oriented communications and push messaging, and they are numbers driven with a short-term focus that coincides with Wall Street's demands. The long run is a quarter, and strategy is how Wall Street bids the price of the stock.

Public interest is an abstraction and in an era of multinational corporations (MNCs), it applies to many publics in many countries at the same time. MNCs leverage the wage and price structures of one country against another to maximise profits. Their views of humanism and freedom are tempered by the opportunities to reap profit in societies where neither are a high priority (e.g., China). Page's view was that of an American nationalist, but we compete today in a global environment where pursuit of wealth allows indifferent treatment of publics that do not have the power or will to remove a company's freedom. MNCs are skilled at using differences between societal expectations and regulations as profitable opportunities.

Consider China. There, pursuit of profit has created factories with low paid workers churning out goods that have made competitive manufacturing in the US and elsewhere unprofitable. What to the US worker is shockingly bad pay is to a Chinese worker better than nothing. A company's pursuit of profit benefits millions of Chinese even as it disadvantages millions of American labourers. MNCs note there is no rule that business must be nationalistic.

We can examine other Page Principles against the same background.

- Tell the truth. Let the public know what's happening and provide an accurate picture of the company's character, ideals and practices.
- Prove it with action. Public perception of an organisation is determined 90 percent by what it does and ten percent by talking.
- Listen to the customer. To serve the company well, understand what the public wants and needs. Keep top decision makers and other employees informed about public reaction to company products, policies and practices.
- Manage for tomorrow. Anticipate public reaction and eliminate practices that create difficulties. Generate goodwill.

— Conduct public relations as if the whole company depends on it. Corporate relations is a management function. No corporate strategy should be implemented without considering its impact on the public. The public relations professional is a policy maker capable of handling a wide range of corporate communications activities.

— Remain calm, patient and good-humored. Lay the groundwork for public relations miracles with consistent, calm and reasoned attention to information and contacts. When a crisis arises, remember that cool heads communicate best.

One can place numbers against these principles, but they would be irrelevant. If the leaders of a company do not have a truth-telling ethic, it takes a law like Sarbanes-Oxley to compel them, but compulsion does not relate to whether a business is successful. Plenty of profitable businesses have lied and will lie and get away with it. Plenty of profitable businesses have ducked responsibilities to act on what they have promised customers and regulators. Plenty of profitable businesses manage for today and not tomorrow.

Many have no public relations arms and the notion of remaining calm, patient and good-humored during a crisis is foreign. They might not engage with the public at all if they can get away with it. When a businessperson or business school student focuses on profit and profit maximisation, relationship and reputation considerations have little bearing. Is it any wonder the two sides cannot talk to one another without translation? Page had an answer for this, but his answer hasn't percolated into any business school text. Here is an excerpted letter he wrote to the executives of the Continental Oil Company. The Continental Oil Company was chartered by public authority on the assumption that it would serve the public's needs for petroleum products.

The theory was that its self-interest would insure its activity and competition would keep its products and services and its prices satisfactory. That is still the main basis of Continental's relation to the public. It is still a fact that the company was set up under pubic authority to benefit the public, and public authority can at any time limit its functions, its methods or abolish it altogether. "So we, like all other companies, live by public approval and roughly speaking, the more approval you have the better you live. This is the fundamental reason for seeking public approval. The fundamental way of getting it is to deserve it. As a management function, public relations encompasses the following:

Anticipating, analysing and interpreting public opinion, attitudes, and issues that might impact, for good or ill, the operations and plans of the organisation. The free flow of information to aid informed decision-making, integrity, honesty and accuracy in all communication and openness that builds trust and credibility. But in pursuit of profit, free flow of information is beside the point and often deleterious to the completion of economic transactions. Business need only supply sufficient information to complete a transaction - e.g. basic characteristics and price of a product or service. It is often the case that missing information includes limitations on products or services that make them useless to the buyer.

In other words, deception is part of the transaction. Deceptive techniques of marketing are and will be used as long as there are buyers and sellers. The Latin phrase, "Caveat Emptor (Let the buyer beware)" applies in an environment where making a profit is proof of business success.

Recent incidents such as paying journalist commentators to promote political agenda is close to what early publicists PR did when they paid reporters and editors to write favorably about products and services. The notion of arms-length persuasion of the news media and conferred credibility of impartial journalistic evaluation were later developments in modern PR. They are principles that many businesspersons dislike because they lack control over communications outcomes. That is why advertising and promotion command the lion's share of expenditures, even though advertising agencies have moved close to a time-billing model and away from commissions. The largest PR accounts today appear to be in marketing as well and consist more of push messaging - publicity placement and promotion -than of mutual adaptation between a company and its publics.

Relationship and reputation management must remain a concern for any business that plans to be around for the long term, but it might not be a priority where profit is the difference between success and failure. That said, there is room for idealism that PR practitioners bring to the corporate environment. Practitioners, however, must be prepared to defend their principles and to suffer defeat. The tougher the competitive environment, the more likely it is that rulebending will occur and PR principles will be less important, unless the CEO personally takes up the cause. Few companies today have the sanctuary of a monopoly in which to focus on relationships as much or more than on return.

5

PUBLIC RELATION IMPLICATIONS

Public relations can be examined from a variety of frameworks, including systems, critical, and rhetorical perspectives. The rhetorical approach focuses on how public relations is engaged in the construction of messages and meanings that are intended to influence key publics important to an organisation.

Rhetorical theory encompasses a wide range of approaches, including argumentation, advocacy and persuasion, corporate communication, dialectics and discourse, dramatism and storytelling, information, organising, public opinion, and reputation management. Yet, none of these approaches represents a comprehensive foundation for fully understanding the processes or consequences of public relations.

Another theoretically rich approach that offers the potential of subsuming and tying together many of these seemingly unrelated approaches involves framing theory. Framing has been used as a paradigm for understanding and investigating communication and related behaviour in a wide range of disciplines. These include psychology, speech communication, organisational decision making, economics, health communication, media studies, and political communication.

Framing theory provides a potentially useful umbrella for examining what occurs in public relations. In addition to a rhetorical approach that focuses on how messages are created, framing is conceptually connected to the underlying psychological processes that people use to examine information, to make judgments, and to draw inferences about the world around them. This linkage is missing in many of the other rhetorical frameworks.

Moreover, framing phenomena operate across levels of analysis, making framing theory applicable at the intrapersonal, interpersonal, group, organisational, interorganisational, and societal levels in which public relations influence attempts operate.

FRAMING

It is important to recognise that public relations work fundamentally involves the construction of social reality. The constructivist approach to communication draws on ideas from the symbolic interactionism school of sociology. Symbolic interactionism rejects attempts to examine human behaviour in terms of instinct, external forces, or the structural-functional explanations that predominated early sociological thinking.

Instead, human behaviour is thought to result from how people interact and their use of symbols to create meaning. Constructionists contend that representations of objects or problems in people's minds vary from the corresponding actual objects or conditions on which they are based. More important, constructionists contend that people act based on these perceptions, or what Lippmann deftly described as "the pictures inside our heads," rather than "objective reality".

Public relations workers have been referred to pejoratively as "imagemakers" and "spin doctors"-labels that only partially portray their important role in constructing social reality. Indeed, public relations counseling involves defining reality for organisations by shaping organisational perspectives about the outside world-a process also termed enactment.

Similarly, outbound public relations communications involve attempts to define reality, at least as it relates to client organisations, for the many publics on whom the organisation depends. This construction process might be dismissed as manipulation. However, because defining reality is the very essence of communication, constructionists would argue that the process is neither inherently good nor bad.

Framing is a critical activity in the construction of social reality because it helps shape the perspectives through which people see the world. Although public relations practitioners commonly refer to framing effective messages in the same way that a builder frames a house from the bottom up, the framing metaphor is better understood as a window or portrait frame drawn around information that delimits the subject matter and, thus, focuses attention on key elements within. Thus, framing involves processes of inclusion and exclusion as well as emphasis. The essence of framing processes with the following:

Framing essentially involves selection and salience. To frame is to select some aspects of perceived reality and make them more salient in the communicating text, in such a way as to promote a particular problem definition, causal interpretation, moral evaluation and/or treatment recommendation for the item described.

Frames, then, define problems – determine what a causal agent is doing and costs and benefits, usually measured in terms of cultural values; diagnose causes – identify the forces creating the problem; make moral judgments – evaluate causal agents and their effects; and suggest remedies – offer and justify treatments for the problem and predict their likely effects.

Implicitly, framing plays an integral role in public relations. If public relations is defined as the process of establishing and maintaining mutually beneficial relations between an organisation and publics onwhomit depends, the establishment of common frames of reference about topics or issues of mutual concern is a necessary condition for effective relations to be established.

As a property of a message, a frame limits or defines the message's meaning by shaping the inferences that individuals make about the message. Frames reflect judgments made by message creators or framers. Some frames represent alternative valencing of information (i.e., putting information in either a positive or negative light, or valence framing).

Other frames involve the simple alternative phrasing of terms (semantic framing). The most complex form of framing is storytelling (story framing). Story framing involves:

— Selecting key themes or ideas that are the focus of the message and

— Incorporating a variety of storytelling or narrative techniques that support that theme.

Framing can be evidenced in a series of structures within a message. These include syntactical structures, stable patterns of arranging words and phrases in a text; script structures, the orderly sequencing of events in a text in a predictable or expected pattern; thematic structures, the presence of propositions or hypotheses that explain the relations between elements within a text-including the presence of words such as "because," "since," and "so"; and rhetorical structures that subtly suggest how a text should be interpreted. Rhetorical devices can include metaphors and similes, familiar exemplars and illustrations, provocative language and descriptors, catchphrases, and visual imagery.

Framing operates by biasing the cognitive processing of information by individuals. At least two mechanisms to explain the process are found in the literature. One suggestion is that framing operates by providing contextual cues that guide decision making and inferences drawn by message audiences. Drawing on their earlier work on the concept, Kahneman and Tversky suggested that the simple positive-versus-negative framing of a decision operates as a cognitive heuristic or rule-of-thumb that guides decisions in situations involving uncertainty or risk.

Negative reactance to losses or risks is consistent with other findings in the impression formation literature that suggest negative information is weightedmoreheavily than positive information and is more attention-getting. It is also consistent with motivational theories that people act to protect themselves. More recent evidence for this heuristic explanation was provide. The elaboration likelihood model to suggest that negative framing might serve as a peripheral cue in processing. Specifically, negative framing might prompt people to think more about a message.

This finding is consistent with research that suggests that message framing effects vary by level of involvement. The second mechanism through which framing operates is priming. Knowledge is thought to be organised in human memory in cognitive structures or schemas, which operate as constraints on the arrangement and interpretation of situations and events. Alternatively, schemas have been conceptualised as categories (hierarchial structures), as prototypes (idealised representations of objects within particular classes), and as scripts (expected scenarios for events).

Although the schematic organisation of memory has been challenged, the notion jibes with at least three of the major models that describe memory in terms of associative networks, storage bins, and distributed memory models. Regardless of the specific model, researchers agree that schematic processing entails people using association and expectation to make inferences about events and to impute meaning not manifested in the message itself.

Significantly, some researchers use "frame" synonymously with schema to delimit which memory nodes are associated with a particular topic in memory. Framing affects cognitive processing by selectively influencing which memory nodes, or sets of memory traces organised as schemas, are activated to interpret a particular message. Priming effects can be conscious, such as when a person purposefully uses message cues to attempt to retrieve stored knowledge from memory.

Priming effects also can be unconscious or automatic, such as when a person categorises a topic or message during the pre-attention phase of processing and then processes information using rules that are considered appropriate in the situation.

Framing Models

Although a theoretically rich and useful concept, framing suffers from a lack of coherent definition. An exhaustive literature search suggests the existence of more than 1,000 citations about framing in the academic literature. Framing has been adopted as a textual, psychological, and socio-political construct.

Depending on the circumstances, the meaning of framing varies based on the research question, the level of analysis, or the underlying psychological process of interest. Framing's ostensible weakness also is one of the concept's inherent strengths. Framing's emphasis on providing context within which information is presented and processed allows framing to be applied across a broad spectrum of communication situations.

An examination of the literature across disciplines suggests at least seven models of framing that have potential application to public relations. By examining these alternative conceptualisations, it is possible for researchers and practitioners to understand the usefulness of the framing concept, to apply it in practice, and to pursue a systematic research agenda about framing as it might be applied to public relations. The seven models involve the framing of situations, attributes, choices, actions, issues, responsibility, and news.

Framing of Situations

Researchers from anthropology and sociology were the first to examine communication using a framing paradigm. Their legacy of using framing to describe how reality is constructed through language and the structure of interactions among people can be labeled as relational or situational framing. A psychological frame as "a spatial and temporal bounding of a set of interactive messages".

The participants' understanding of the interaction in which they engage – including their roles and the rules to be followed – operate as a form of metacommunication. The notion and described framing as "the definition of a situation built up in accordance with principles of organisation that govern events – at least social ones – and our subjective involvement in them".

A frame as a "schemata of interpretation" that provides a context for understanding information and enables individuals to "locate, perceive, identify and label". Of these, three of the most important were keying, bringing into focus particular aspects of everyday life by recreating past interactions; anchoring, the rooting of ideas in deeper frames of meaning; and fabrication, the recasting of certain dimensions of experience so they are made salient within a situation or interaction.

Two of the most important research domains relevant to public relations in which situation framing has been investigated involve organisational behaviour and negotiation. Framing as the process by which managers at all levels attempt to impose their version of reality on situations. Normative framing has facilitated acceptance of once-disdained business practices, such as hostile takeovers. In the same way, organisational framing (i.e., the use of frames by organisations in its discourse) has been used to examine contemporary problems.

Examples include sexual exploitation and concealment of sexual harassment. Economists similarly have employed framing concepts. Social norms, or unconscious rules of social exchange behaviour, have been used to contrast actions in different types of economic systems. They suggested the business contexts in which individuals work provide important cues that frame understanding of problems and lead to distinct behaviours.

In the negotiation arena, bargaining is defined through the processes of framing and reframing that occur throughout the deliberations. Other researchers have examined the linguistic patterns used by bargainers to frame negotiations and the critical role of mediators as framers and reframers of issues.

Framing of Attributes

Separate from defining and describing overall situations found in everyday life and literature, a second and distinct form of framing involves the framing of attributes (i.e., the characterisation of objects, events, and people). Semantic framing is used to focus on particular attributes that might be flattering or derogatory and, thus, be advantageous or disadvantageous to message sponsors in persuasive communications.

Consumer behaviour researchers are the most active in attribute framing research and use the term in at least four distinct ways. Picture framing describes ads in which captions accompany a photo and are used to prime the cognitive processing of visuals by calling attention to particular attributes depicted. Problem framing refers to the deliberations used by decision makers, particularly novices, to structure a preference judgment task.

Advertising has been shown to influence judgments by altering key aspects of the decision process by refocusing consumer attention away from certain attributes or choice rules in favor of others, thus defining (framing) the criteria on which decisions should be made and the schema that should be used. Advertising framing of product experience, drawing on William D. Wells's notion of transformational advertising, suggests that promotional messages transform how the consumer perceives and judges the subsequent consumption of a product.

Finally, experience – frames – advertising effects have been identified. These involve how a consumer's prior experiences and satisfaction using a particular product bias the salience of particular product attributes in a commercial message and, thus, influence the criteria used to judge messages and featured products. Product positioning is another term commonly used by marketers to describe attribute framing. Positioning as the "act of designing a company's offerings and image so they occupy a meaningful and distinctive competitive position in the customer's mind".

Positioning heightens product expectations and enables consumers to differentiate people, objects, and brands. Although they do not use the term "schema". People rank products and brands using "little ladders" in their heads; the ladders are product categories, and the ladder rungs represent brands. Framing also has been used to describe alternative presentation of product claims or attributes.

Alternatives examined include whether the product is described (framed) based on price versus benefits, product connections to political concerns (pro-environmental "green marketing") versus instrumental qualities, and the alternate anchoring (framing) of price references. Finally, framing also is central to research about comparative advertising that examines claims made about a particular product's attributes relative to others in the same category.

Attribute framing has received increased attention in media studies from Maxwell McCombs and his colleagues. Media are effective in not only raising the salience of particular topics, issues, or objects but also can create specific knowledge of attributes related to issues and people, such as political candidates. The media's ability to create general top-of-mind salience about a topic is known as agenda-setting.

McCombs labeled the media's ability also to frame attributes as second-order agenda setting or frame setting. The extension of the familiar description of agenda-setting thus suggests, although media are not necessarily effective in telling people what to think, media can be strikingly effective in telling people what to think about - and how to think about it.

Beyond marketing and communications, attribute framing has been used by economists to explain economic behaviours. The theory of institutional framing suggests that perceptions of fairness (i.e., an attribute of an institution involving whether it deals fairly with others) accounts for aberrations not explained by standard economic models that emphasise self-interest. Other economists reject classical notions of economics that presume people use a single absolute zero-base as the starting point for making economic decisions.

Instead, people are thought to use multiple reference points in decision making; each of these reference points represents a distinct frame of reference that is used to assess attributes or values when making comparisons. Finally, still other neoclassical economists reject the notion that people are rational in making decisions and only seek economic benefits (utilities).

These economists contend that nonrational economic behaviour can be explained by the fact that individuals seek a variety of different benefits (utilities) and that any of these can dominate decision making at a given time and can thus focus judgments on different attributes. In examining research in psychology related to decision making. Attribute framing involves individuals making evaluations of particular attributes of an object. They assume no risk is involved.

In general, attribute framing relies on semantic differences related to making what is fundamentally the same choice, such as a describing beef as "75% lean" or "25% fat". Attribute framing also can involve effects from alternative descriptions of the success-failure rate of a particular procedure (i.e., whether results emphasise a 60% success rate or a 40% failure rate), or win-loss rates (i.e., whether a team won 30 games or lost 20 games). Positive framing of attributes consistently leads to more favorable evaluations of objects and attributes than negative framing.

Framing of Risky Choices

A third important area of framing for public relations involves the framing of risky choices, wherein individuals must not merely evaluate attributes but must make a choice between two independent options when some level of uncertainty or risk is present. (The framing of risky choices can be distinguished from framing where no independent choice is at issue and only one course of action is involved.

The framing of choices is one of the most extensively researched areas of framing, based on the classical work of psychologists Daniel Kahneman and Amos Tversky. A frame as a decision maker's perception of "the acts, outcomes, and contingencies associated with a particular choice". In particular, they argued that human decision making is inherently nonrationale because the prospect of a loss has a far greater impact on decision making than does the prospect of an equivalent gain.

In developing their prospect theory of decision making, the psychologists began with an expected-value model wherein it was assumed, in a linear fashion, that an individual who finds Rs. 1 would happy and that a person who finds Rs. 100 should be 100 times happier. Conversely, they theorised that a person who loses Rs. 100 should be proportionately more distressed than a person who loses only Rs. 1.

Instead, the researchers discovered an S-shaped curve of responses wherein the prospect of greater gains was perceived as less valuable but that the prospect of even a modest loss far outweighed the prospect of a comparable modest gain. People tend to avoid risks when a choice is stated in terms of gains but will take greater risks when choices are stated in terms of losses. Prospect theory's revelations about the predominant influence of loss-prevention has been a topic of ongoing interest among researchers. Although a variety of moderating factors have been suggested, framing effect has largely withstood testing.

Most studies of prospect theory have involved hypothetical, experimental situations. Original question involving how people would respond to an Asian disease. However, research about the framing of choices has been conducted in a wide range of applied domains as well. For example, health communicators have found patients are willing to select greater risks if the decision means saving a life or reducing suffering.

The same phenomenon has been observed among health care professionals. Findings consistent with prospect theory are reported in the negotiation literature. Mediators have been found to favor bargainers who frame issues in terms of losses rather than gains. Mediators also propose settlements of higher value when both parties frame decisions in loss terms.

A programme of research on the effects of framing on negotiations spearheaded by Margaret Neale suggested that how a negotiator's role is framed influences the negotiator's task orientation to seek the greatest possible concessions, that positive framing of a negotiator's self-confidence leads to more concessions, and that framing can moderate the effectiveness of even expert negotiators.

Organisational behaviour researchers have found that individuals in businesses are willing to take greater risks to avoid losses rather than to seek gains. Marketers similarly have used prospect theory to examine purchasing risk behaviour. Finally, economists have examined the influence of framing on the risk tolerances among auditors and financial planners and the effect of framing persuasive messages related to taxpayer compliance.

However, the effect varies by the domain of the choice. For example, People are more willing to take risks to save human lives than to preserve public property or save personal money. This is consistent with research in health communication that suggests that the context of the decision influences willingness to take risks.

Framing of Actions

Closely aligned to prospect theory's emphasis on the influence of framing gains versus losses, other research related to decision making has focused on the best way to describe action that might be undertaken by individuals to achieve a desired goal. This idea can be labeled framing of actions.

The framing of attributes involves focusing attention on inherent qualities of an object, and whereas the framing of risky choices focuses on willingness of individuals to take risks, framing of actions focuses on persuasive attempts to maximise cooperation in which no independent options or choices are involved. For persuasive communicators, the concern is how to frame actions necessary to achieve compliance with a desired goal.

A familiar example illustrates the idea: Some universities allow students to pay tuition early in a lump sum or to pay a slightly higher amount in installments. Assuming that a university wanted to improve its cash flow, the desired action of paying money earlier can be framed as a discount (a gain), whereas the installment plan might be framed as a surcharge (a loss). The two explanations are different semantically, but the options are the same.

Framing of actions is similar to purevalence framing as used by economists and to goal framing. The latter researchers explain that positive action (goal) framing involves focusing attention on obtaining a positive consequence (gain), whereas the negative frame focuses attention on avoiding the negative consequence (loss) resulting from not taking a particular action.

A specific applied domain in which action framing is especially pertinent is in the effort by health practitioners to promote healthy behaviours and communicate the dangers of risky behaviours. Framing studies have been conducted in the context of preventing automobile accidents, cancer, Downs syndrome, HIV, sexually transmitted diseases, and weight control problems, among others.

People's willingness to engage in particular health-related actions have been shown to be influenced by how risks and alternatives are framed, although various moderating factors have also been suggested. Research in economic psychology similarly suggests that individuals differentially will make choices about the same personal benefits derived from society as a whole, based on whether the issue was framed as an action involving a social dilemma or a public goods problem.

Findings from research involving the framing of actions is somewhat similar to the results obtained in research obtained in the framing of risky choices but differs from findings pertaining to the framing of attributes. Framing of actions in terms of negative consequences appears to have greater persuasive impact than framing that emphasises positive consequences or gains.

Positively framed messages might be more persuasive when people engage in little detailed processing of messages and that negative framing of actions only applies when people engage in higher levels of cognitive elaboration. Although the presence of negatively framed arguments might prompt more elaborate message processing, the effects also might be moderated by an individual's expectations about the type of framing found in a persuasive message.

The effect is also moderated by an individual's perception of self-efficacy (i.e., whether a person believes that following a particular action will lead to the desired outcome). Individuals with high levels of self-efficacy are less inclined to engage in effortful processing, in which case positive and negative frames are equally persuasive. Other factors that influence the framing of actions include the level of consumer expertise and the presence or absence of social interaction.

Framing of Issues

Framing has received increased attention among sociologists and others as a way to examine alternative interpretations of social reality. This approach can be labeled the framing of issues. An issue is a dispute between two or more parties, usually over the allocation of resources or the treatment or portrayal of groups in society. Issues frequently result in extensive public discussion and frequently require resolution within a public policy forum, such as a legislature or the courts.

Issues are the bases around which publics are organised and public opinion is formed Issues can be constructed by as few as two individuals but also can emerge at the group, organisation, interorganisational, or societal levels. At the heart of most issues is the question of interpretation. Disputants involved in an issue often vie to have their preferred interpretation predominate so that others will see the dispute from a perspective similar to their own (i.e., using similar schemas).

Framing has been employed as a tool for analysing public debates on issues and as the focus of still other research in the arenas of negotiation and bargaining.

Legal theorists also have recognised the importance of effective issue framing as a key strategy in persuasively communicating with jurors. Organisational behaviour researchers have employed issues framing as variable to understand why and how decisions are made and actions are undertaken.

Applications range from ethical decision making to emergency response planning and employment practices. Framing similarly has been used to examine people's judgments of the fairness of allocation of economic resources. Studies in economics have focused on issues such as income equity, tax equity, willingness to pay for public goods, and social conflicts pertaining to environmental and public health risks.

Framing plays a pivotal role in defining social problems and the attendant moral actions in dealing with them. Investigators outside media studies have used a variety of methods to study the framing of controversies involving politics, gender rights, race, property rights, the threat of religious cults, and the marginalisation of various groups in postmodern society.

In a similar vein, public health issues have been shown to be dramatically influenced by the way they are represented. For example, AIDS has been framed alternatively as a disease involving "high-risk groups" and resulting from "risky practices". Sympathy for AIDS victims varies considerably depending on whether AIDS is described as a disease affecting hemophiliacs, intravenous drug users, or homosexuals.

Social researchers who adopt a constructionist approach argue that social problems are best understood as issues that are constructed by claim makers. Advocates for issues engage in a process of agenda-building that involves mobilizing support, building coalitions, manipulating symbols, and actively seeking publicity in public media. Agenda-building involves pushing issues from the arenas of public discussion, onto the media agenda and ultimately to the public policy agenda, in which issues and social problems can receive official acknowledgment, validation, and the fullest possible hearing.

However, not all issues fully attain public visibility. Among factors that determine the success of issue advocates is the limited carrying capacity of the system as well as the frame enterprise and the effectiveness of frame sponsorship by issue advocates. This process also can be conceptualised as frame building. Framing plays an integral part in the process of agenda-building as advocates attempt to communicate with members of affected or sympathetic groups, either directly or indirectly using the media.

In the latter case, social identification theory suggests the goal is to signal uninvolved group members about how they should think or act in regard to an issue. Frames operate in this definitional process as "devices embedded in political discourse, invented and employed by political elites, often with an eye toward advancing their own interests or ideologies and intended to make favorable interpretations".

In doing so, claims makers try to influence which schematic representations of issue are invoked by politicians and media workers and, most important, by media audiences.Social movement organisations have theorised extensively about the importance of framing. Snow and Social movements engage in three distinct framing processes. Diagnostic framing involves the identification of an event or aspect of social life as problematic or in need of alteration.

Prognostic framing proposes a solution to the diagnosed problem and outlines what needs to be done.

Finally, motivational framing represents a call to action as well as the rationale forengagingin ameliorative or corrective action. Elsewhere, the researchers define framing as a device for mobilisation wherein groups attempt to create linkages amongotherwise disparate individuals through a process of frame alignment.

Four strategies identified by the researchers are frame bridging, frame amplification (clarification and crystallisation of beliefs and values held by followers), frame extension (reaching out to include other constituencies), and frame transformation (in which frames are altered in the wake of changing conditions).

Framing of Responsibility

Beyond matters of definition, most issues and social problems entail questions of cause and responsibility (i.e., who should be credited or blamed for events). Whether because of instinct or experience or for self-protection, individuals engage in what Heider termed "intuitive factor analysis" to understand why events happen. Attribution of an event to either personal or environmental factors determines the extent to which an individual is held responsible.

However, the attribution of responsibility does not always reflect the objective facts of a situation accurately and can be distorted based on how events are described. This accounts for yet another type of framing relevant to public relations, the framing of responsibility. Attribution processes, or how humans explain events and human behaviour, have received extensive attention from psychologists.

Theory of causal attribution identified three distinct types of attributions: to an actor, to the object or entity acted on, or to the environment or circumstances in which an event occurs. When individuals have multiple opportunities to observe events, Kelley suggested that attributions are based on patterns of covariation involving three factors: distinctiveness, the extent to which different entities evoke similar behaviour; consensus, the extent to which different actors behave in a similar way; and consistency over time and modality, the extent to which the behaviour is similar in different contexts.

In situations in which only one opportunity to observe is possible. People will tend to give less credence to the role of a given cause if other plausible explanations are also present. Similarly, his argumentation principle suggested that facilitative causal explanations of events are judged more plausible than inhibitory casual explanations if both are considered.

Later attribution research suggests that actions can be labeled (framed) as controlled or uncontrolled, internally or externally originated, or as a result of stable or unstable conditions within a person. Ability, for example, represents an explanation for success that combines internal and stable factors within an individual. Luck or fate, on the other hand, entails external, unstable factors. Attribution processes are easily biased as a result of a variety of factors. These include a lack of effort to find the "best" explanation, the salience of alternative explanations, prior knowledge and extant schemas, and personal needs and motivations.

Fundamental attribution error refers to the tendency to attribute other people's behaviour to stable personality factors or dispositions rather than situations or external causes. Actor-observer bias is the tendency to attribute other people's behaviours to stable dispositions, whereas people attribute their own behaviour to situational factors. Self-serving bias involves self-attributions of success or failure: People tend to attribute their own successes to stable dispositions and their failures to situational factors.

Personal control bias suggests that humans assign blame for disastrous occurrences in proportion to the perceived severity of the consequences.

Finally, the just-world hypothesis suggests evaluations of a victim's suffering become increasingly negative to the degree that the victim's suffering is seen as unjustified. All these ideas suggest that the way an event is portrayed can lead to different conclusions about responsibility. Although some events occur for unidentifiable reasons (so-called "acts of God"), most individuals are unwilling or unable to accept such a simple explanation.

Most people seek to identify the cause and assign responsibility. Americans frame issues to portray the overall social system as fundamentally sound and prefer to attribute problems to corrupt, inept, or irresponsible individuals. The result is to ignore systemic problems related to social organisation or societal resources available to deal with a problem. As a result, events that might have been prevented through intervention simply are dismissed later as accidents due to human error.

Various problems – AIDS, alcoholism, child abuse, cigarette addiction, drug abuse, and overeating – have been framed as problems of individuals rather than society. The solution often involves the medicalisation of problems, wherein emphasis is placed on treatment of individuals rather than on prevention or elimination of the root causes at the societal level.

Efforts to assign responsibility for issues and social problems is referred to as diagnostic framing – a process that can be at work among individuals as well as groups. Diagnostic framing plays a central role in investigative journalism. News workers often begin with a single incident and then work inductively to identify other cases or individuals who might be affected. After sensing the inherent dramatic values in a story, investigative reporters conceptualise a story by placing it within a broader context through framing.

Stories are identified as part of a particular investigative genre and typified as an example of a particular well-known problem, such as political corruption, corporate exploitation, or government waste and inefficiency. As the drama unfolds further, roles inevitably are assigned to victims and villains. Attribution processes are evident in the way that media subtly frame stories and assign responsibility.

News coverage is predominated by the episodic framing of stories to exclusion of thematic framing. Episodic framing involves storytelling from the perspective of people and individual events. Audiences are believed to be more interested in people and more responsive to portrayals involving concrete events and actions (episodes). By contrast, media engage in comparatively little thematic framing, where stories are told more broadly from a societal perspective using abstract concepts instead of case studies or exemplars.

An unintended consequence of the preponderance of episodic framing is that audiences feel absolved of responsibility for social problems because responsibility is so readily attributed to the people portrayed in the news, whether or not the newsmakers depicted are culpable. The desire to attribute responsibility has lead to an emphasis on victimisation in modern society, although stories about victims suffering at the hands of villains can be found in literature across cultures over the centuries.

The seemingly natural tendency is for victims to attribute responsibility for their misfortunes to misdeeds of others, rather than assume any responsibility for their own plight. Although production-of-action is one element of responsibility, causality and responsibility are distinct concepts. Responsibility can subsume causality but also can incorporate notions of legal accountability and moral accountability. Significantly, legal culpability is addressed in courts of law, whereas moral accountability is debated and framed in the court of public opinion.

Framing of News

The final model of framing relevant to public relations deals with news framing (i.e., how news stories are portrayed or framed by the media in an effort to explain complex or abstract ideas in familiar, culturally resonating terms).

Framing has received considerable attention in the past decade as an approach to understanding news processes and effects, although the role of public relations as sources in news framing has been largely overlooked. To recognise the integral role that framing plays in news gathering by media workers and news processing by audiences. News workers use frames to construct social reality for audiences and thus give meaning to words and images.

News workers as "symbol handlers" who use frame selectivity to shape the way news is defined using dominant social frames. The ideas that appear in news are best understood as media packages that feature a central organising idea for events and employ various symbolic or framing devices that support the main idea of the story. The task of media workers thus is to arrange random events into a meaningful, organised interpretive package.

Later media theorists have paid increased attention to framing as an alternative formulation of issues such as bias and objectivity. Hackett observed framing is not necessarily a conscious process on the part of journalists but is the result of their unconscious assumptions about the social world. Although frames are not unique to journalism, they are central to journalistic work and serve as "mental maps" that can be activated quickly and can reduce journalists' efforts.

The ability of media to raise the salience of attributes and to frame values. Strong effects that go beyond simple agenda-setting. Separately, considerable discussion has ensued about how to measure framing effects and role of framing as both dependent and independent variables in media research.

The topics of news framing studies have spanned a wide range of social problems, including abortion, America's "drug problem", Cold War criminals, child mistreatment, fathers' rights, labour strikes, and welfare. Framing also has provided a useful perspective from which to examine portrayals of occupational groups such as artists, as well as ethnic minorities.

The media's portrayal of scientific issues and processes, including issues such as climate change, cold fusion, ozone depletion, and memory recovery. Of particular interest has been the role of framing in the reporting about risk. Specific topics examined within the domain of risk communications involve environmental issues and disputes as well as issues pertaining to public health and the availability of public health services.

6

TYPOLOGY OF THE PUBLIC RELATIONS BEHAVIOUR

A general theory of the public relations (PR) behaviour of organisations remains an elusive goal of scholars. Attempts such as four models developed by the researchers fall short of a PR theory of orga nisational behaviour, since most organisations practice each of the models at different times. For this reason, it is not yet possible to classify organisations by their practice of PR, to predict the type of PR an organisation will use, or to explain the effect of different types of public relations on organisational performance.

Some of the organisational scientists believe theories of organisational behaviour must begin with a "classification of the species" in order to identify homogenous populations within the species about which falsifiable hypotheses can be formed and tested. A preliminary classification system, or typology, of public relations behaviour based on a new construct called public relations orientation is shown in Figure 1. The constructed types presented here describe what type of organisation practises what type of public relations, and what organisation level outcomes may be expected from pursuing public relations strategy through a given type.

Classification is an essential prerequisite to good science because it identifies homogeneous populations within the larger species (in this case, organisations) about which falsifiable hypotheses can be formed. By specifying the diversity inherent in the species called "organisations" organisational behaviour can be explained and predicted. Types are "constructed" by ordering or synthesising a complex set of variables for comparing and measuring objectively probable phenomena. Typologies meet the criteria for theory building because they contain constructs or variables on which a theoretical system can be built, they specify relationships between the constructs, that is, they generate hypotheses, and they are empirically testable.

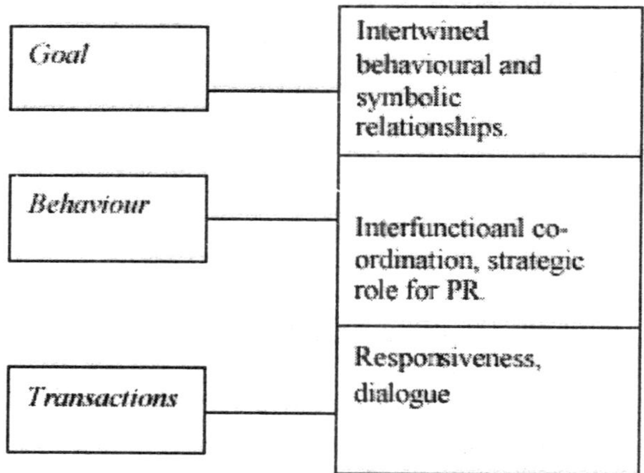

Figure 1: The Dimensions of Public Relations Orientation

Good typologies should specify the dimensions of the type and how they are measured and describe the logic underlying the configuration of dimensions. Additional criteria include terminological clarity, essentiality, extensiveness, inclusivity, systematisation, power, theoretical productivity, logic, and prescriptive utility

Mitnick. With these guidelines in mind, begin the task of constructing a typology of the public relations behaviour of organisations, based on our construct, "public relations orientation".

PUBLIC RELATIONS ORIENTATION (PRO)

The term "orientation" is used to describe the possible philosophical stances of an organisation towards public relations (Figure 1). Orientation involves

a) A specific goal (direction),

b) A description of the way one acts as a consequence of the goal, and

c) The response one adopts when dealing with things external to one's self.

Thus, an orientation can be described in terms of the characteristics of the goal, the goal directed behaviour, and the transactions with the environment and parties threatening or enabling the achievement of the goal (stakeholders). Explication of public relations orientation is based on five dimensions grouped under the three categories of goal, behaviour and transactions. Each of these dimensions will now be described and its underlying variables deconstructed. Each is also generally measured as "high- low".

Goal Dimension of Public Relations

The goal dimension of public relations has two axes: the quest for positive images (symbolic relationships) and the quest for substantive behavioural relationships between organisations and publics. PR people can set short term objectives to improve symbolic relationships with publics, but over the long term public relations should "examine behavioural relationships with publics relationships that directly affect the ... ability to accomplish organisational goals".

High PRO occurs when behavioural and symbolic aspects of relationships are "intertwined". When they are separated, public relations practitioners offer little value because "they suggest that the problems in relationships with publics can be solved using the proper message disseminated through publicity or media relations to change an image of an organisation". The disconnection of symbolic relationships from behavioural relationships represents low PRO. The two sub-dimensions, each specified as high or low, lead to four possible cells, which form the foundation of the proposed PRO typology (Figure 2). The four cells are high behavioural relationships/high symbolic relationships (HBR-HSR), named "integrated"; low behavioural relationship/high symbolic relationship (LBR-HSR), named "promotional"; high behavioural relationship/low symbolic relationship (HBRLSR), named "technical"; and low behavioural relationship/low symbolic relationship (LBRLSR), named "restricted".

Public Relations Behaviour

The PR behaviour category is based on two dimensions: interfunctional co-ordination, and a strategic role for public relations. These dimensions are considered the foundation of effective public relations behaviour of organisations.

Interfunctional Co-ordination: Constraints on information collection and dissemination, which is call interfunctional coordination, limit public relations effectiveness. Interfunctional coordination is a term borrowed from the marketing literature, to indicate the integration of efforts by all parts of the organisation to achieve the PR goal (integrated symbolic and behavioural relationships). It includes the systematic generation, analysis and dissemination of intelligence across functional boundaries about relationships with publics or stakeholders.

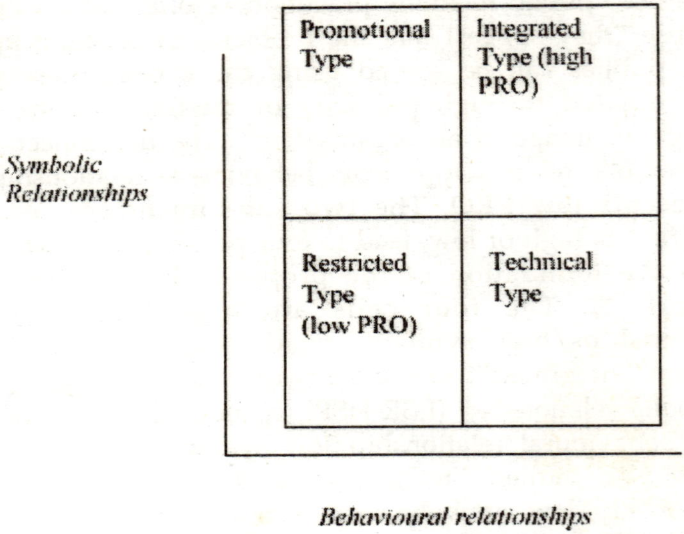

Symbolic Relationships

Promotional Type	Integrated Type (high PRO)
Restricted Type (low PRO)	Technical Type

Behavioural relationships

Figure 2: A Typology of the Public Relations Behaviour of Organisations

Strategic Role: Scholars have identified the presence of a strategic role for public relations as a requirement of public relations "excellence" and its lack as a constraint on public relations effectiveness.

Transactions with Environment

The third category of PRO dimensions is the transactions of the organisation with actors in its environment (publics) who threaten or enable achievement of the public relations goal (high, intertwined symbolic and behavioural relationships). This category has two dimensions, responsiveness to stakeholders and a dialogic approach to stakeholder relationships.

Responsiveness

Responsiveness is implicit in much of the public relations literature. However, the concept of responsiveness adopted here is based on the results of the grounded theory study. The responsiveness atom has two axes, one being the intensity of activity ranging from "do little" to "do much", the other being the nature of activity, ranging from "adversarial" to "collaborative". The twoby-two structure of this dimension leads to four possible cells, which conform closely to the responsiveness modes. The do- much/collaborative cell is named "proactive" (lead the industry); the dolittle/ collaborative cell is named "accommodative" (be progressive); the domuch/ adversarial cell is named "reactive" (fight all the way); and the do-little/reactive cell is named "defensive" (do only what is required).

Dialogic Approach

A dialogue process is necessary to fully and accurately identify stakeholder needs and to negotiate effective responses. Dialogue is a precondition for ethical public relations. Dialogue in this model is composed of respectful attitudes towards the dialogic partner, mutual agreement about the structural attributes of communication, and mutual satisfaction with the rules of communication. Effective, ethical dialogue also requires openness and a willingness to disclose information that is critical to the relationship.

Integrated PR Organisation

In the integrated public relations organisation, the public relations goal synthesises high symbolic and high behavioural relationships with publics. The public relations function has a strategic, managerial role and its manager is most likely to generate valuable outcomes for the organisation. The organisation effectively utilises public relations intelligence to adapt itself to its changing stakeholder environment, which may be both complex and dynamic. The integrated PR organisation is proactive in that it actively seeks collaborative solutions to conflict with publics or stakeholders.

Dialogue and openness are key relationship maintenance strategies, providing an ethical framework for decision making. This organisation is likely to hold a symmetrical worldview for public relations and is more likely than the other types to use symmetrical public relations strategies, although mixed mode strategies will be used. Among the four types, this organisation is most likely to practice "excellent" public relations. The integrated public relations type is expected to be most frequently associated with the "analyser" strategic type. The analyser organisation tries to exploit new product and market opportunities (requiring attention to symbolic relationships that can signal quality or other attributes to prospective customers) while maintaining a firm base of traditional products and customers (requiring attention to behavioural relationships aimed at improving customer loyalty, repeat purchase and so on).

The ability of public relations managers to develop measurable, strategic public relations goals and strategies that support the overall business goals will lead to influence within the dominant coalition. The major problem faced by public relations managers in integrated organisations is the tension between the need for innovation in relating to new or changing publics and the need for efficiency without staleness in relating to traditional publics. When executed well, the organisation level public relations outcomes for this organisation are likely to include a good reputation, legitimacy (license to operate), and reduced conflict with stakeholders.

Promotional PR Organisation

The promotional PR organisation pursues high symbolic relationships with publics, but does not place the same emphasis on behavioural relationships. Therefore, the organisation's actions do not always match its rhetoric. While intensely active, the organisation's asymmetrical worldview for public relations leads to behaviour aimed at persuading publics that it is right, which is an adversarial, rather than a collaborative, type of responsiveness. Interfunctional co-ordination is moderate as the type of PR information exchanged within the organisation relates only to the organisation's ability to promote itself and not the full stakeholder environment.

In the promotional public relations organisation, public relations may contribute to image making strategy, but not to overall organisation strategy. The organisation selectively attends to stakeholder groups important to its image, such as customers. It does not seek dialogue, although it may seek feedback in order to more scientifically persuade its publics that it is right. It is moderately open, insofar as is required to promote itself to various publics. The correlates of the promotional type are, therefore, an assymetrical worldview for public relations and a managerial role for public relations.

The managerial role is posited because the manager is likely to have control of an adequate budget for promotio ns and use research to ascertain the effectiveness of promotional programmes. The promotional type of organisation may be most closely associated with the Miles and Snow "prospector" strategic type. The prospector is continually modifying its productmarket domain to take advantage of perceived opportunities and therefore has a high requirement for both marketing and promotions. Its requirement for speed to market means that attention to long term collaborative relationships with stakeholders takes a back seat to the requirements for symbolic, image making activity. Creative approaches to public relations will flourish in this organisation when the top communicator is able to enact a managerial role.

However, the inherent inefficiencies of the prospector's rapidly changing, diverse operations may be a trap for the public relations function, which typically requires a long term focus for maximum impact. The organisation may have an active PR department and be well recognised because of its intense image making activity, but its failure to attend to substantive behavioural relationships puts it at risk of stakeholder cynicism, and ultimately, loss of reputation.

Technical PR Organisation

The technical PR organisation pays a lot of attention to maintaining good stakeholder relationships but places little emphasis on image, believing that actions speak louder than words. The organisation is not well known except among those it has a direct relationship with. Long term relationships with key publics are likely to be collaborative rather than adversarial; for example, the organisation may be a supplier of customised components to long term customers in a stable industry. While responsive, the organisation takes little initiative and routine communications predominate. PR interfunctional co-ordination is low because public relations generates little valuable intelligence for the organisation.

In this organisation, the worldview for public relations is technical, and public relations plays a technical role rather than a strategic role. Public relations will use little or no research, set output rather than outcome goals, and make little contribution to the achievement of business goals. The transactional dimensions of public relations orientatio n, namely responsiveness and dialogue, are moderate because even though public relations has little input, the organisation as a whole has an accommodative approach towards its long standing stakeholders. This organisation is most like the Miles and Snow "defender" type, which has a relatively stable environment, with few changes to its product market domain.

This organisation is focused on efficiency to defend its narrow market domain. Because the product market domain is stable, and public relations enacts a technical role, life for the public relations staff is predictable and routine. Changes in its business environment or business strategy put this type at risk unless it develops a proactive communication plan to keep emerging and existing stakeholders well informed.

Restricted PR Organisation

The restricted PR organisation places little value on either symbolic or behavioural relationships with stakeholders. It is least likely to have a discrete public relations function, thus it is the most restricted organisational environment for public relations. When publics intrude into the operations of the organisation, the response is to do as little as possible (defensive). Because publics are not valued, neither is the public relations function, and all of the dimensions of public relations orientation will be low. If the organisation has a public relations person, the person's tasks are likely to be technical, or even clerical, in nature, such as distribution of statutory reports or product samples.

Such an organisation may be successful with a low public relations orientation if it is has few and undemanding stakeholders. However, low attention to stakeholder relationships is an unsustainable strategy for most organisations. The strategic impotence of the restricted PR type makes it like the "reactor" type defined by Miles and Snow. This type represents a failure of an organisation to use any of the other strategies to adapt to its product market environment. Miles and Snow suggest that reactors, which are inherently unstable, fail to adapt to their environment. A public relations manager is unlikely to be able to perform well in this organisation.

Thus far, described a new construct called public relations orientation and developed a typology of the public relations behaviour of organisations based on its dimensions. The typology meets Mitnick's essential criteria for a good typology because it includes all relevant entities (all organisations whether they have a public relations function, or not), captures important features of public relations behaviour in a systematic way and has a clear logic.

TYPOLOGY OF POWER

A powerful typology is one that subsumes other typologies. Several typologies have been developed in public relations theory. For example, worldviews for public relations have been identified as symmetrical and asymmetrical. Our integrated type is symmetrical, while the other three types are asymmetrical. The technical type, however, may well emulate the technical worldview. Public relations roles have been typified in the literature as managerial and technical. Managerial roles are more likely to predominate in our integrated and promotional types, and technical roles are expected to prevail in our technical type. Our restricted type may not have a discrete public relations function.

Another PR typology is the four models of public relations. Each of the models may be practised in all of our types except the restricted type, although symmetrical public relations will be practised more in the integrated type than in any of the others. Use of the models in each type is more likely to vary by intensity. In other words, the integrated type uses all the models more than the promotional type, and the promotional type uses all the models more than the technical type. Public relations environments have also been classified as complex/ simple and turbulent/static. Relating the public relations types to the Miles and Snow typology addresses aspects of the product market environment. However, public relations is also concerned with publics in the non market, or social and political environment. The addition of non market environmental variables to the types suggests a further research direction.

Finally, structure of the public relations department has been classified in relation to the Hage-Hull typology with limited success. The typology addresses structure via linkage to the Miles & Snow typology, which is based on the variables of structure, strategy and process. However, more remains to be explained about the contribution of the structure of public relations to organisational performance. Nevertheless, even at this preliminary stage of development, a typology based on public relations orientation has considerable power.

Each of the types can be considered a midrange theory that explains how public relations works within a particular type of organisation. However, types are most useful in theory development when they are treated as independent variables in a grand theoretical assertion, that is, that variation in the types predicts something. By linking our typology with the Miles and Snow typology, suggesting that variation in the public relations types explains some variance in organisational performance. The pathway by which public relations contributes to performance is by managing behavioural and symbolic relationships with publics.

Symbolic relationships may influence reputation, which in turn impacts performance. Behavioural relationships may reduce the level of conflict, which contributes to performance by lowering costs. Behavioural relationships may also engender co-operative behaviour from publics, which leads to outcomes such as legitimacy (license to operate) and loyalty. Thus, the types contribute to a general theory of the public relations behaviour of organisations, by hypothesising how each type contributes to performance (or not).

The multi-dimensional construct, public relations orientation, clearly has prescriptive utility as managers can use it as an organisational diagnostic, to make changes to the public relations mission, behaviour or stakeholder transactions. Prescriptive utility also arises because each type relies on a public relations strategy that is more or less likely to produce particular outcomes, such as reputation or reduced conflict with stakeholders.

7

RISK COMMUNICATION GUIDELINES

People often fail to effectively communicate due to a lack of clear communications goals and key messages to support them. Setting such goals and identifying support messages are decisions that should be made prior to the issuing of any public comment and are especially important in a crisis. A communications goal of "educating the public on the complexities of bioterrorism and preparing them for any eventuality" is not realistic; informing the public of the problem and specific dangers, providing guidance on appropriate responses, and easing concerns are achievable goals.

Messages in support of these goals must also be direct and effectively speak to the audience. A discussion of statistical probabilities and how they translate into a "relatively minimal-risk scenario for the average citizen" might be fine for scientists, but for the general public such a discussion will only confuse the issue and fail to meet the goals of informing and easing concerns. If the risk is low, say, "the risk to the public is low."

a) Goal #1: Ease public concern
   — The risk is low.
   — The illness is treatable.

   — It is not easily contracted.
   — Symptoms are easily recognised.

b) Goal #2: Give guidance on how to respond
   — Take these precautions.
   — If possibly exposed, contact physician.
   — If symptomatic, contact physician.
   — Note possible symptoms in others.

Once goals and messages have been established, the challenge becomes one of delivery and ensuring that messages are heard and goals are met. The method for accomplishing this is what has come to be known as being "on message" and is, essentially, a form of artful repetition. If the goal is to ease concern and the message in support of that goal is, "the risk to the public is low," that message should be clearly stated at the outset and returned to as often as possible:

"I want to begin by first saying that the risk to the public is very low...."

"As I said a moment ago, the risk to the public is low...."

"That's an important question, but before I answer it I want to again stress that the fact remains that the risk to the public is low."

"Before I close I want to remind everyone that the risk is low."

— Raise your points often enough that your audience leaves with a clear understanding of the message you wanted them to hear.

— Take opportunities to begin or end statements with a reiteration of your message.

— Don't be so repetitious with a single message that you appear to be trying to convince people of something that isn't true.

— Don't repeat your messages word-for-word every time you answer a question.

Another aspect of staying on message is to exercise some control over the conversation you are having, be it an interview, press conference, or questions from an audience. Don't allow the conversation to be led down paths that are not pertinent to your goals or message-no matter how persistent the questioner might be in pursuing a line of inquiry.

Sound and thoughtful risk communication can assist public officials in preventing ineffective, fear-driven, and potentially damaging public responses to serious crises such as unusual disease outbreaks and bioterrorism. Moreover, appropriate risk communication procedures foster the trust and confidence that are vital in a crisis situation. There are steps public officials can take in advance of any incident to better prepare communities, risk managers, government spokespersons, public health officials, the news media, physicians, and hospital personnel to respond to the challenges of managing such crises.

Plan for communicating to the public and the news media by asking yourself the following questions:

— What information is crucial to convey in initial messages in order to prompt appropriate public responses after a crisis situation?

— What are the messages to be delivered prior to, during, and after an incident?

— What are the obstacles to effective communications and how can they be minimised?

— What are the opportunities for effective communications and how can they be maximised?

— What questions can we anticipate from the public in these risk situations?

— What are the news media's responsibilities and how can you help reporters meet them?

The cardinal rule of risk communication is the same as that for emergency medicine: first do no harm. A threatening or actual crisis often poses a volatile equation of public action and reaction. This destabilised information environment makes it very important that you give thought to what it is you are about to say before making any public comment-be it a 30-second statement to a news person or a 30-minute news conference to a roomful of media representatives.

In preparing for this speaking opportunity:

— Assess the environment into which you are introducing information. Gain a sense of the public's general attitude toward the situation and tailor your presentation accordingly. Are they worried and in need of reassurance? Are they sanguine and in need of a warning? Are they angry and in need of calming?

— Review your remarks to gauge the probable impact that your words will have on the situation and adjust them as necessary; e.g., are you using words, like "crisis," "life-threatening," or "extremely" and can other, less dramatic words be substituted?

— Understand your audience. If it is a reporter, appreciate the demands and constraints under which reporters work and recognise the risks those constraints pose to you as a communicator.

— Don't speak unless you are comfortable doing so. Most communications mistakes are made by those who are not prepared to speak but feel compelled to do so anyway. If confronted with a demand for a quick answer, have the confidence to say, "I would like to answer that question later."

— Don't assume you're not in need of help, and don't be shy about asking for it. Always take advantage of whatever professional communications support is available to you. If you have access to a public affairs office, use it. You can also hire a local public relations consultant or ask a corporate public relations executive to volunteer to help you meet your challenges.

— Watch, read, and listen to the news; analyse how it is presented; critique the communications skills of others; learn from their successes as well as from their mistakes.

Provide Accurate and Quick Information

In a risk communications situation there is a constant tension between providing accurate information and providing information quickly. Both demands pose dangers. To wait for all information to be complete and verified before releasing it to the public can create an information vacuum that will almost certainly be filled with rumor and speculation. To release information that has not been double-checked and which turns out to be inaccurate, however, runs the risk of misleading the public and undermining your credibility as a spokesperson.

The best way to address this challenge is to establish regular briefings with the media (in person or via conference call) at which time all information can be delivered, explained, and updated. If information is an estimation, it can be presented as such and its preliminary nature stressed to the media. This approach, combined with the fact that the information will be updated in the near term, keeps information in its proper context and prevents it from becoming etched in stone before it is fully and finally verified. It also keeps the media attentive to the changing nature of the issue with which they are dealing and attuned to the need for maintaining contact with you in order to keep their stories accurate and up to date.

a) If you hold regular briefings, do so at a time that meets the deadline needs of the media.
b) Be prepared to explain the meaning behind evolving information; e.g., "Concerning the increase in this number, that is a reflection of our having increased the number of people tested, it is not a reflection of an increase in what we have always recognised as the population-wide average."
c) If you suspect that the next information update will drastically change a story, give reporters a sense that such may be the case.
d) Always provide statistics and key information to the media in written form.
e) Always know how information was gathered and conclusions reached.

SCIENTIFIC AND TECHNICAL INFORMATION

Scientific information will be more useful to the audience and greater communication success will be achieved if the information provided is relevant and easily understood. To help audiences understand the issues, create well-targeted messages. Also be sure to use clear, non-technical language to discuss risks and other specific information indicating the nature, form, severity, or magnitude of the risk. Ways to better communicate complex scientific or technical information:

a) Use consistent names and other terms throughout a crisis situation (e.g., switching from parts per million to parts per billion can result in alarm because the higher numbers may be noticed, but not the unit of measure).

b) Avoid acronyms and jargon (e.g., excess lifetime cancer risk) and provide careful definitions in advance.

c) Carefully consider what types of visuals the news media may want, be sure all information is explained fully, and use these visuals to clarify and support key communications points.

d) Answer not only the question, "How much?", but also the question "Will it hurt me?" to ensure the information is relevant.

e) Use familiar frames of reference to explain how much, how big or how small and try to create a mental picture of such measures as "parts per billion" or "tons per day."

Numeric analogies-e.g., the U.S. produces enough garbage in a day to fill 100 football fields 14 feet deep-are much more meaningful to average listeners than talking about 250,000 tons of garbage per day. However, examples should not be trite or condescending or overly dramatic. Take the time to develop meaningful examples and calculations. Indicate the level of certainty of your information, for example, "We are 95% certain, but we are conducting more studies to improve the accuracy."

Scientific Uncertainty

Recognising and admitting uncertainty is simply the reality of most risk communication situations. Unfortunately, scientific uncertainty is a complicating point in satisfying the public's demand for reliable and meaningful information for many hazards and risks. Public health officials frequently face the dilemma of having to acknowledge and explain uncertainty to a public that thinks scientific findings are precise, repeatable, and reliable. Moreover, the public often associates correlation and association as being the same as causality. As a result, officials often face the additional task of trying to explain the data's limitations and uncertainties.

If information is not known or not available, the best thing to do is to honestly admit it. Saying "I don't know" is an acceptable response and can actually build credibility. Audiences need to be provided as much information as possible to help them understand that uncertainty is part of the process and that the answers available now may not be the final answers. If an audience demands 100% certainty, they are more than likely questioning the underlying values and process, not the science. Try to identify the real concerns behind the demand for certainty and address them.

Because the risk communication process is so deeply embedded in broader social issues, communicators are faced with many barriers. A key barrier is the term "risk" itself, how it's measured, described, and ultimately perceived. Interested parties perceive risk differently, and people do not believe that all risks are of the same type, size, or importance. The perceptions of risk for the technical and lay audience are often dissimilar. For example, the public health official or scientist uses a one-in-a-million comparison to convey a specific risk measurement.

Health experts understand this to mean that, given one million persons, there is one person who is at risk. To the non-technical person, however, the one person may be someone they know. The public will often personalise risk with the same conviction that most scientists depersonalise it. Ultimately, the public will decide how much risk is acceptable and their decision will be based on personal factors.

One goal for the public health official should be to educate the public on the level of risk and competing risks. Trying to sell the public on acceptable risk may be difficult because people would prefer to live without any health and environmental concerns. However, by listening to and addressing concerns, the target audience will be better able to understand and, possibly accept, the risk.

Factors Affecting Risk Perception

Perceptions of the magnitude of risk are influenced by factors other than numerical data. Understanding these factors will help you gauge the degree of risk with which your message may be perceived, and assist you as you craft your communications strategy.

Building Trust and Credibility

Your ability to establish constructive communication will be determined, in large part, by whether your audiences perceive you to be trustworthy and believable. Consider how they form their judgments and perceptions. Key factors in assessing trust and credibility are: empathy and caring; competence and expertise; honesty and openness; and dedication and commitment. Five Rules for Building Trust and Credibility:

1. *Accept and involve the public as a partner*: Work with and for the public to inform, dispel misinformation and, to every degree possible, allay fears and concerns.
2. *Appreciate the public's specific concerns*: Statistics and probabilities don't necessarily answer all questions. Be sensitive to people's fears and worries on a human level. Your position does not preclude your acknowledging the sadness of an illness, injury, or death. Do not overstate or dwell on tragedy, but do empathise with the public and provide answers that respect their humanity.

3. *Be honest and open*: Once lost, trust and credibility are almost impossible to regain. Never mislead the public by lying or failing to provide information that is important to their understanding of issues.
4. *Work with other credible sources*: Conflicts and disagreements among organisations and credible spokespersons create confusion and breed distrust. Coordinate your information and communications efforts with those of other legitimate parties. Unless you are assured that the subject to be discussed will be tightly confined to your area of expertise, it is usually not best to serve as the sole spokesperson on an issue. Crisis situations have multiple facets and raise a range of questions. Having people on hand who can answer those questions facilitates and speeds the communications process and better ensures that informational voids don't develop. Identify those colleagues and other officials and experts who can speak to the issues that are most likely to be raised and rely on their help when it's needed.
5. *Meet the needs of the media*: Never refuse to work with the media. The media's role is to inform the public, which will be done with or without your assistance. Work with the media to ensure that the information they are providing the public is as accurate and enlightening as possible. Conflicting information, particularly when it comes from equally trusted sources, creates confusion and erodes confidence. Know what other spokespersons intend to say and support their messages.

If something that you don't agree with is said, or if wrong information is presented, do not publicly contradict the statement or disagree with the spokesperson. Resolve the matter in private and present the new information to the public as a simple correction or clarification of a previous statement and not as one opinion having prevailed over another.

Avoiding Pitfalls

Abstractions: Use examples, stories, and analogies to make your point. Don't assume there is a common understanding between you and your audience (even when you are using stories and analogies to make your point).

Attacks: Respond to issues, not to people. Strive to end debates, not further them. Don't respond to an attack with an attack of your own.

Attitude/Non-verbal messages: Remain calm, attentive and polite. Adopt a relaxed, neutral physical stance. Don't let your feelings interfere with your ability to communicate positively. Never convey disgust, frustration, indifference, or smugness. Never lose your temper. Don't allow your body language, your position in the room, or your dress to affect your message.

Blame: Accept your share of responsibility for a problem. Don't try to shift blame or responsibility to others and don't magnify the fault to be found in others in order to deflect criticism or minimise your culpability.

Costs: Focus on the benefits to be derived, not on the costs entailed. If costs are an issue, voice respect for the need for responsible stewardship of public funds. Don't discuss issues in terms of their dollar value, or complain about a lack of funds.

Guarantees: It is better to offer a likelihood, emphasising progress and on-going efforts. Don't make comments like, "There are no guarantees in life."

Humor: Avoid it. If used, direct it at yourself. Don't use it in relation to safety, or health, or in describing risk.

Jargon: Define all technical terms and acronyms. Don't use language that may not be understood by even a portion of your audience.

Length of presentations: Plan, practice and deliver a cogent 15-minute presentation. Don't believe that what you are saying is inherently more interesting than other topics and therefore warrants more time. By the same token, don't end your remarks after 15 minutes if there are important audience questions in need of answering.

Negative sllegations: Refute allegations succinctly. Don't repeat allegations or refer to them in ways that give them credibility.

Negative words and phrases: Use positive or neutral terms. Don't cite national problems, or make highlycharged analogies, e.g., "This is not Love Canal."

"Off the record": Always assume everything. You say and do is part of the public record. Don't make side comments or "confidential" remarks. (the rule is: never say anything that you are not willing to see printed on the front page of a newspaper.)

Personal identity: Speak for the organisation. Use the pronoun "we." Don't give the impression that you, alone, are the authority on the issues being raised or the sole decision-maker. Never disagree with the organisation you are representing, e.g., "personally, i don't agree," or "speaking for myself...," or "if it were me...."

Promises: it is better to state your willingness to try. Promise only what you can deliver. Don't make promises you can't keep and never make a promise on behalf of someone else.

Reliance on words alone: use visuals and hand-outs to emphasise key points. Don't rely entirely on the spoken word to explain your point.

Speculation: stick to the facts of what has, is, and will be done. Don't speculate on what could be done, or on what might happen, or on possible outcomes other than the intended one(s), or about worst case scenarios.

Statistics: Use them to illuminate larger points and to emphasise trends and achievements. Don't make them the focus of your remarks, or overuse them.

Technical details and data: Focus on empathy, efforts and results. Don't try to fully inform and educate audiences on the minutia of issues.

Managing Hostile Situations

Issues of health and safety can arouse strong emotions, including anger and hostility. Dealing ineffectively with hostility can erode trust and credibility. Remember, though, public hostility is usually directed at you as a representative of an organisation, not you as an individual, so don't take it personally.

Diffusing anger and hostility

— Acknowledge the existence of hostility. The worst thing you can do is pretend it's not there.

— Practice self-management. Send the message that you are in control.

— Control your apprehension. Anxiety undercuts confidence, concentration, and momentum.

— Be prepared. Practice your presentation and anticipated questions and answers.

— Listen. Recognise people's frustrations-communicate empathy and caring.

— Assume a listening posture. Use eye contact.

— Answer questions thoughtfully. Turn negatives into positives and bridge back to your messages.

COMMUNICATION WITH MEDIA

The media are a primary means for communicating with the public. Forming positive relationships with journalists is crucial to your communications success. As a matter of ethics, journalists will not allow "news" to be defined for them. The advantage of this is clear: neither government, nor business, nor anyone can control the news for their own purposes. The disadvantage, however, is that there are no absolutes in what constitutes news and issues that are important to some, or many, may never be addressed by the media because they fail to meet what is, essentially, an indefinable standard for attention.

Journalists strive to answer six key questions in their stories: who, when, where, what, how, and why. All the information they gather somehow informs, explains, or elaborates on those six issues and often raises doubts or breeds confusion when the facts of a news story are juxtaposed, e.g., "Government sources said there was no immediate danger; however, local hospitals have instituted emergency measures." The facts of a story also become somewhat relative when, in upholding the principle of fairness, journalists balance one set of facts with other facts or opinions, e.g., "Government sources said there was no immediate danger, but one expert disagreed."

Although presented in an effort to further illuminate the subject and present the reader with perspectives that help provide a truer picture of the whole story, it poses a relativism that can lead to public confusion and mistrust. All of these imponderables of reporting and news coverage make communicating with and through the news media an imprecise endeavor. What you say may not be what is determined to be news. How you say it may lead to confused and confusing reports and misinterpretations. Whatever you say is likely to be balanced against opinions that are different than yours.

Guidance on Dealing with Facts

a) Be sure of your facts.

b) Be able to cite sources and key statistics, making sure they add meaningful support to your message (this could be three key statistics or thirty, but be careful not to overwhelm your message with statistics).

c) Have information available in fact sheets and other concise informational documents specifically prepared for the media's use.

d) Familiarise yourself with information and opinions that are contrary to your points and positions and be able to answer the questions they raise.

Space and time place critical demands and limitations on a journalist's work. First is the need just to fill space and time. A newspaper has never failed to publish or a newscast failed to air because there was no news on a given day. The news business demands that every day there be enough news to fill a certain number of pages or minutes, and that demand is always met no matter the relative importance of the news to be covered on a "slow news day." This demand makes for a great deal of reporting on issues and individuals that may seem trivial.

This is often the case with stories that dominate the news over a period of time. The need for continuing coverage of a major story usually leads to coverage of aspects of the story that are less important but still may be of interest to the public; e.g., profiles of individuals involved in the story, different reactions to the story, etc. The more you can provide the media with substantive information that allows for substantive reporting, the less the chance that reporting will stray into less important areas. Parallel to the media's challenge of having to fill space, television and radio news face the problem of having too little time for available news.

Competition for time with advertisers and the standard broadcast features of sports and weather means that the very longest stories will only be a few minutes in duration and the shortest as brief as 20 seconds. While newspapers don't suffer such extreme limitations, they, too, find space a finite resource and will frequently cut stories to fit the size of the day's "news hole" (the space left to fill in a newspaper after advertising and standard news and entertainment features are laid out). Effective communication comes not in fighting these limitations, but in adapting to them.

If the time that is given you is limited-as it most certainly will be with television or radio-make sure that your primary message gets delivered within the time allotted. If you are given more time to expound and expand on your message-as you might be in a newspaper interview-use it, but do not abuse it by overexplaining your points or straying into areas of comment that do not add to a better understanding of the topic.

Guidance on working within space and time constraints are;

a) Know your communications goals and supporting messages.

b) Arrange them in a hierarchy of importance and develop brief (20-30 second) statements that explain each one.

c) Practice delivering your statements in front of a mirror.

d) Closely observe how others are quoted by the media, particularly in radio and television "sound bites." Refine your statements so that your messages can be delivered via such brief quotes.

What many people see as journalists' antagonistic attitudes toward public officials is often simply part of the basic conflict that exists between someone who has information and someone who wants it. A reporter's job is to gain as much pertinent information as possible to answer the six key questions entailed in every news story. It's a job that demands skepticism and requires that few statements be taken at face value. Be patient, open, and honest in fielding questions, no matter how hostile they may seem.

If you run into a conflict with the media, keep it in perspective and don't take it personally. Be sensitive to the full context of reporters' questions. Are they confused by the information you're giving them, or have they gotten it wrong? Do they seem overly skeptical, frustrated, or even angry? If so, do not shrug it off. Journalists' emotions affect their reporting. It's your responsibility to remain patient and work with them to overcome those negatives.

a) Reporters are not your enemies, but neither are they your friends. They owe you nothing and you should not expect any more from them than fairness and courtesy.

b) Under no circumstances allow professional disagreements to turn into personal arguments.

c) Don't hold grudges.

The adage is: Never say anything today that you don't want to see on the front page of The New York Times tomorrow. If you say to a reporter, "Well, between you and me, the guy is an idiot," you should expect to see it in a story... and you won't look good. If you call the reporter to complain, you should expect to see your complaint in a follow-up story... and you still won't look good. If you get angry and stop talking to the reporter, you can expect to see that, too, reflected in a story... and you'll look even worse.

Guidance for Interview Situations

a) Consider yourself the reporter's guest.

b) Be courteous and patient when answering (and re-answering) questions.

c) Adopt the attitude of assisting the reporter in doing his or her job.

d) If you tell a reporter you'll get back to him or her, do it!

e) Never be too casual in your conversation. Remember, whatever you say could end up in a news story (even if you think it's off the record). If you make an ill-considered comment, and it ends up in the newspaper, it is not the reporter's fault. It's yours.

Using the full advantages of an interview

— LISTEN to the question being asked, THINK about your answer, and always try to deliver and redeliver your message(s).

— Discuss what you know, not what you think.

— Do not express personal opinions. If you are compelled to violate this dictate, make certain that you are very clear in distinguishing opinions from official positions and policies.

— Don't speculate or try to respond to questions to which you don't know the answer.

— Don't show off. This is not the time to display an impressive vocabulary or present the full extent of your intellect and knowledge. Talk as you might to your neighbor.

— Do not worry about looking stupid. If you are confused by a question, say so. If you say something that's wrong, or misstate a fact, don't defend it, admit your error.

— Don't engage in off-the-record discussions.

As a matter of normal conversation, we always speculate, hypothesise, and offer opinions. But an interview is not a normal conversation. Be careful of what you say. And don't start thinking that just because a reporter happens to be asking you questions, your opinions are worth more than the messages you're supposed to be delivering.

Planning and Preparations

Much of the success of effective risk communications is predicated on the amount of work that goes into planning and preparing for a crisis event. What information needs to be in place, who makes decisions, who gives orders, and who follows them? What are the procedures for carrying out response initiatives? A crisis is not the time to begin thinking about these questions. In fact, it's the worst time to do so.

Risk communication efforts should receive the same preparation as any other possible emergency. Lists of contacts with addresses and phone numbers should be drawn up (and updated regularly) and fact sheets and background materials should be prepared. The tools and information needed to communicate fully and effectively when a crisis erupts have to be readily accessible. And, most importantly, an agreed-to protocol for action must be in place. Some guidance for planning and preparations are;

a) Form a risk communications team.

b) Designate a team leader and assign responsibilities to team members.

c) Develop a risk communications protocol.

— Who decides when a crisis exists, what are each team member's responsibilities?

— Who speaks to the media/public on what subjects and at whose direction?

d) Develop and maintain lists.

— Primary contacts/experts for key offices and issue areas.

— Secondary contacts/experts for key offices and issue areas.

— Media lists. (A media list is a list of print, broadcast, and electronic media that will allow your communications team to identify every possible national, regional, and local outlet and analyse its potential value for reaching your target audiences.)

e) Consider logistics.

— Where would a press briefing be held? Is it easily accessible? Is the room large enough? Will it accommodate media needs for sound quality and sufficient power? Will speakers need chairs, tables, or podiums?

f) Identify information needs and develop appropriate fact sheets and background materials.

Hundreds of questions-some good, some trivial, some odd-emerge when a news story is breaking. The more questions that can be anticipated and answered ahead of time in a fact sheet the better. This is especially true for information regarding high visibility public health issues such as might occur in a bioterrorist event. Readily available information on these issues will help keep misinformation to a minimum.

Do's and Don'ts in an Interview

Before

Do

— Ask who will be conducting the interview.

— Ask which subjects they want to cover.

— Caution the interviewer on the limits of your knowledge.

— Inquire about the format and duration.

— Ask who else will be interviewed.

— Suggest other interviewees.

— Prepare and practice.

Don't

— Allow yourself to be interviewed on a topic outside of your expertise.

— Tell the news organisation which reporter you prefer. (You don't run the newspaper and you don't get to dictate who gets assigned what stories.)

— Request that specific questions be asked.

— Declare certain subjects out of bounds for discussion. (By declaring that you won't discuss certain things you only invite interest in those things and appear to have something to hide, which makes the subject even more interesting.)

— Ask that your remarks not be edited or that you be allowed to review an article before it is published. (It is an insult to the ability and integrity of the reporter and the editor; again, you don't run the newspaper.)

— Try to dictate who should and should not be interviewed.

— Be over-confident or become overly familiar or comfortable with your interviewer.

During

Do

— Be honest and accurate.

— Deliver and re-deliver your key message(s).

— State your conclusions first, then provide supporting data.

— Be forthcoming to the extent you decide beforehand.

— Offer to get information you don't have.

— Stress the facts.

— Give a reason if you can't discuss a subject.

— Correct mistakes by stating you would like an opportunity to clarify.

— Assume that microphones and recording equipment are turned on.

Don't

— Lie or try to cloud the truth.

— Improvise or dwell on negative allegations.

— Raise issues you don't want to see in the story.

— Answer questions off the top of your head.

— Speculate, guess, assume or hypothesise.

— Speak for others.

— Say "no comment."

— Be led into other areas of discussion.

— Demand that an answer you have given not be used. If you say it, you have to live with it. You can ask that it not be used and explain why you would prefer that it not be used, but you can't demand anything... and if the reporter chooses to use it, there's little you can do.

After

Do

— Remember you are still on the record.

— Be helpful. Volunteer to get information. Be available.

— Respect deadlines and deliver whatever additional information you said you would deliver.

— Follow-up to see if any additional questions have emerged.

— Watch for and read the resulting report.

— Ignore minor reporting errors that don't affect the point of the story.

— Call the reporter to politely point out if there are inaccuracies that do effect the point of the story.

Don't

— Assume an interview is over or that recording equipment is turned off.

— Refuse to talk further.

— Ask, "How did I do?"

— Ask to review the story before publication or broadcast.

— Complain to the reporter's boss first.

In a crisis

Do

— Plan now.

— Respond quickly-the first 24 hours are critical.

— Respond straightforwardly.

— Be accurate.

— Strive to reassure as well as alert and inform your audience.

Don't

— Assume "it will never happen here."

— Allow your issues to be defined by someone else.

— Think that refusing to discuss a story will allay public concerns or prevent people from seeking, and finding, information-accurate or not-elsewhere.

Correcting the Mistakes

If substantive inaccuracies (i.e., inaccuracies that have the potential to further a crisis or problem) occur, you should move very quickly to correct them. Remember-the longer misinformation remains viable in the information environment, the more difficult it becomes to correct. In this situation,

a) Move quickly to correct them.

b) Keep the level of your response appropriate to the level of the problem.

   — Overreacting to an isolated mistake will only attract attention to the very problem you are trying to correct. (A single yet important error of fact in a newspaper article would probably be best dealt with by a polite call to the reporter who made the error.)

   — Underreacting to widely reported information that is not correct will only allow for a compounding of the error. (In this case a public statement or even a news conference might be most in order.)

c) If a damaging rumor is confined to a small audience, correct it within that group, don't create a major public event.

d) If a damaging rumor is widely known and spreading-making it difficult for you to reach your communications goals-you should move aggressively and very publicly to correct it.

e) When squelching a rumor, try to anticipate how the rumor might evolve in response to your efforts and be as thorough as you can in closing off possible avenues of future, similar rumors.

For example, if the rumor is that, "The police are planning to evacuate the downtown area," your response should be clear and unequivocal: "There are NO plans to evacuate any section of the city," so that the details of the rumor can't change into something like-"The National Guard is planning to evacuate the city." Be careful, too, that your comments don't leave the wrong impression and are not open to interpretation. In the above example, for instance, care should be taken to ensure that the statement does not generate the headline, "Officials Concede City Lacks Evacuation Plan." Such a headline could be avoided by adding a statement that further dispels the rumor by clarifying the evacuation issue. For example, "There are no plans to evacuate any section of the city. We have a long-standing emergency preparedness plan in place, and if it were to be activated, the public would be given notice immediately by the Mayor."

EFFECTS OF PERSONAL STRENGTHS AND WEEKNESSE

Individual styles and talents affect communications performance; and while thought and preparation will improve the presentation skills of everyone, they will not correct all deficiencies. Assess your strengths and weaknesses.

a) If you tend to an academic presentation style, work to present information in more human terms.

— If you would be more prone to say: "As you'll see by the data, the incidence of occurrence of this particular event is, statistically speaking, relatively low and tends to remain isolated particularly when compared to similar events noted in the appendix of the document provided you."

— Try saying something along the lines of: "The data show that these kinds of events are rare. They usually affect few groups of people, and don't recur."

b) If you have a rhetorical style, work to include substantive supporting data in your presentation.

— If you would be more prone to say: "Our challenge is to address these issues on a human scale that recognises and strives to preserve an individual's health and quality of life."

— Try saying something along the lines of: "We want to deal with the quality of life issues involved here. Based on the research, that means getting people checked, identifying those affected, which will be approximately one in a million people, and getting them treatment. The statistics show that if we can do that, we'll keep xx percent of people well, and effectively treat xx percent of those few who do become ill."

This is not an attempt to achieve a personal makeover. Don't try to become a great orator or a professorial lecturer. Simply think about how you present information, or ask someone you know well how they think you present information, and see if you can identify ways to improve your style. But don't become so self-conscious of how you present information that it interferes with delivering your messages.

a) If you are uncomfortable in a large group or news conference setting, try to arrange for smaller interview sessions (although take care to provide the same information to each reporter).

b) If you are uncomfortable with one-on-one interviews, include a colleague or staff member in the interview whose strengths will make up for your weaknesses.

PRESENTATION IN A PUBLIC MEETINGS

What you do and how you do it will affect your audiences' perceptions of you, your organisation, and the information you are providing. Prepare and present effectively.

a) Before the meeting knoe your audience:
   - Who are they, where are they from?
   - What are their interests and concerns?
   - What are their likely perceptions and biases?
   - Will they be receptive or resistant or even hostile?

b) Prepare your presentation:
   - Develop a strong introduction.
   - Develop a maximum of three key messages.
   - Assemble your supporting data.
   - Prepare audiovisual aids.
   - Prepare for answering questions.
   - Practice.

How to Start a Presentation

A strong opening presentation sets a tone for the meeting and is crucial in attempting to establish trust and build credibility. Its elements include the following:

a) Introduction
   - A statement of personal concern

- A statement of organisational commitment and intent
- A statement of purpose and a plan for the meeting

b) Key messages

- A maximum of three take-home points
- Information to support the key messages

c) Conclusion

- A summarising statement

Introduction

Remember that perceived empathy is a vital factor in establishing trust and building credibility and it is assessed by your audience in the first 30 seconds. Include the following in your introduction:

a) Statement of personal concern, e.g., "I can see by the number of people here tonight that you are as concerned about this issue as I am."

b) Statement of organisational intent, e.g., "I am committed to protecting the health and safety of the public. The Mayor and his staff have been involved with this community for a long time and want to work with the community on this issue."

c) Statement of purpose and plan for the meeting.

Key messages

The key messages are points you want your public to have in mind after the meeting. They should address central issues, and be short and concise, e.g., "We have performed extensive tests over the past week which have failed to find any evidence that X remains in the building. It is now safe to return there." To develop your key messages:

a) *Brainstorm*: Think freely and jot down all pieces of information you wish to communicate.

b) *Select key messages*: Identify the most important ideas. Repeat the process until your list is down to three items.

c) *Identify supporting data*: Review your brainstorming ideas and background materials for information that provides support to your key messages.

Conclusion

a) Restate verbatim your key messages.

b) Add a future action statement: What is your organisation going to do about this problem in the short term? Long term?

Presentation Aids

Audiovisual aids can make your messages easier to understand. People are more likely to remember a point if they have a visual association with the words. More guidance in preparing quality presentations can be found in the book "Loud and Clear: How to Prepare and Deliver Effective Business and Technical Presentations". Some aids to consider: charts, illustrations, diagrams, glossaries, maps, posters, photographs, video/motion pictures, Microsoft PowerPoint (or equivalent) presentations, lists, fact sheets.

Effective visual aids:

— Are able to stand alone.

— Illustrate a key concept.

— Support only one major idea.

— Use pictures or graphics rather than words whenever possible.

— Conform to six words per line maximum, ten lines per visual maximum.

— Feature short phrases or key words.

— Highlight important points with colour or contrast.

— Represent facts accurately.

— Are carefully made-neat, clear, and uncluttered.

— Have impact.

If you use presentation aids be careful not to overdo it. When planning, practicing, and conducting a presentation, consider:

— *Attire/grooming*: Dress as your audience would expect you to at your place of work or perhaps slightly less formally.

— *Distractions*: Avoid repetitive gestures such as constant throat-clearing, checking your watch, jingling keys or change, and pacing. Take a breath and relax.

— *Enunciation/pronunciation*: Speak distinctly

— *And correctly*: Be careful with unfamiliar words. Spell And define terms as appropriate, but don't be Pedantic.

— *Facial expressions/eye contact*: Eye contact is Most crucial. Your mouth, eyes, forehead, and eyebrows also communicate. Try not to fidget, glance around or lick your lips.

— *Gestures*: Gestures can enhance or detract from your communication. Be aware of yours and make sure they are appropriate, but don't be so worried about not using your hands that you make a poor presentation.

— *Pace/rhythm/pitch*: Vary your tempo. Speak slowly to emphasise key messages, pause for emphasis, vary your voice pattern and length of phrases. Avoid repeating such words as "ok," "like," "not," "uh," and "you know."

— *Posture*: Posture communicates attitude. Try to have a straight stance with legs slightly apart. Don't slouch, but don't be rigid.

— *Volume*: The intensity of your voice reflects your confidence, competence, and openness. Watch your audience for feedback. Adjust to your surroundings. Don't make your audience strain to hear you but don't shout at them either.

How to Answer Questions

As with presentations, your responses to individuals' questions and concerns will affect your success. Prepare and practice. Consider how to answer questions in general and how to respond to specific inquiries.

— *Be Prepared*: If you know your subject and your audience, most questions can be anticipated.

— *Track Your Key Messages:* Use your responses as opportunities to reemphasise your key messages.

— *Keep Your Answers Short and Focused:* Your answer should be less than 2 minutes long.

— *Practice Self-Management.* Listen: Be confident and factual. Control your emotions.

— *Speak and Act with Integrity:* Tell the truth. If you don't know, say so. Follow up as promised. If you are unsure of a question, repeat or paraphrase it to be certain of the meaning.

The discussion of issues surrounding a news event is not confined to official sources or to a single forum. News, comment, analysis, and opinion from innumerable voices enter the information environment by way of newspapers (as news, editorials, opinion articles, letters to the editor), television and radio (as news, in special reports, and through talk shows), and dozens of other sources such as speeches, newsletters, and web sites.

The appearance of information that is related to your issues of concern is an opportunity for you to lend your voice to that particular discussion. Look for ways to insert yourself into the debate surrounding your issues and don't be shy about availing yourself of those opportunities. A newspaper article might give you the chance to author an opinion article or a letter to the editor that would further address the issue. Speaking before a local civic group is another means of delivering your message. And appearing on local talk radio programmes is an excellent way to extend the reach and impact of your messages.

You can do:

— Submit letters to the editors of local newspapers. Contact your local newspaper to find out how to submit an opinion article.

— Call in to local talk radio programmes when pertinent topics are being discussed.

— Contact local talk-radio producers to solicit an invitation to appear on their programmes.

— Contact local civic groups to solicit speaking opportunities.

— If you give a speech, contact local news outlets and ask them to cover your presentation.

— Contact local television news producers to explore ways they can cover your issues.

8

PUBLIC RELATION INTO WEB DESIGN

On-line communications is strongly nicheoriented, the equivalent of going door-to-door and neighbour-to-neighbour in a grass-roots effort. Electronic commerce continues to intensify, providing a strategic blend of marketing, public relations, and technology. Projections on the expansion of electronic commerce have been consistently understated. The internet has become a communication vehicle that can enable business-toconsumer and business-to-business electronic commerce. Its ease of use has resulted in rapid worldwide expansion.

Over the past five years, electronic commerce has exploded, with a significant technological impact on business strategy. Estimates of current use and expectations for the future vary, but in each case, the actual use continues to exceed expectations. Most major companies have developed a web site presence that aims to boost bottom-line results, raising their awareness level or enhancing customer loyalty. For companies doing business on the Internet, effective web design, an e-commerce strategy, and relationship-building will affect their ability to compete.

It is vital for a company to have an integrated marketing, public relations, and information technology strategy to develop a lasting, value-added presence on-line. Public relations practitioners have found that technology can supplement tasks such as maintaining media lists, analysing media clips, and obtaining immediate feedback on the impact of press releases. Specialisation and targeting continue to be significant trends in public relations, and vast web-based databases support these trends.

Yet, it is not uncommon today for business executives to tout success on the Web, based solely on gross revenues and increased traffic to their web sites. While these two metrics are important indicators of success, the authors contend it is equally important to ascertain that customers are satisfied with their experience on the site, and that future sales are linked to customer trust, loyalty, and community-building.

Relationship – building or humanising the digital experience involves becoming interactive and having an intelligent dialogue with customers – in short, becoming connected to customers in multiple forums: on-line, by phone and direct mail, and with toll-free numbers. Interactivity is a building block that leads to lasting customer relationships.

A relationship on the Web today competes with the handshake and the warm reception that customers are used to receiving in a showroom or retail store. e-commerce marketers can learn from the marketing philosophy of the popular home-shopping TV channels, with their consistently boosted sales over recent years.

Customer relationships in that medium are built entirely on interactivity-toll-free numbers flash on the screen; customers talk with the host; the blinking countdown clock warns viewers of a few minutes left to buy before the item is replaced on the screen; and money-back guarantees are stressed. Information satisfaction contributes to consumer satisfaction, which occurs when the product or service which a firm offers consistently matches consumer expectations.

Of course, many on-line customers fail to hit the buy button before they leave a web site because it does not meet their expectations. Customer satisfaction also depends on relationship-building, finding the customers' shared values and helping them become loyal lifetime customers. Therefore, an effective electronic commerce strategy should match the desired consumer response with the web site design.

The consumer response web site design model was developed to provide a framework for describing the relationship between web site design and a consumer's intention to return to a web site. Here included a public relations dimension, to explain how to build long-term customer relationships. The theoretical basis for the model is explained along with its relationship to information satisfaction.

The model purports that the public relations dimension provides a mechanism to build loyalty and trust and that will result in an increase in information satisfaction. How information technology (IT) and public relations (PR) executives working together on e-commerce strategy can build meaningful long-term relationships with Web customers. IT web site design is enhanced by an integrated public relations strategy, thereby achieving a state in which customers not only return to the web site more often, but also have a more favorable image of the organisation.

WEB SITE DESIGN

Web site design is beginning to mature as a component of

an organisations overall information technology strategy. No longer are organisations racing to develop a web site pressence, but instead must establish lasting relationships with their customers. To accomplish this it is important to establish a relationship between the information satisfaction that a customer perceives from a web site.

Information Satisfaction

Consumer satisfaction occurs when the performance of a product or service matches the consumers' expectations. The concept of information satisfaction, which influences the overall feeling of satisfaction that a consumer experiences when given information about a product or service. The importance of information satisfaction increases when the buyer-seller exchange occurs in an on-line environment through electronic commerce.

The marketing interaction that transpires between business and consumer as the creation of real virtuality. Real virtuality states that users' interactions with electronic environments are enhanced by their cognitive experience, which is created not only by what is seen on the screen but also by the communication of the experience. Therefore, real virtuality is enhanced by the amount of information that is made available on a product or service.

Electronic commerce via the Internet is an enabling technology through which firms can provide customercentric marketing. Sheth, Sisodia, and Sharma (2000) define customer-centric marketing as a strategy that seeks to satisfy the needs of individual customers rather than a mass market. Three reasons underscore the growth in customer-centric marketing. First is concern over the effectiveness of marketing activities by senior management. Second, market diversity increases the consumers' wants and needs.

Third, new technologies have enabled marketers to better meet the needs of individual consumers. The degree to which people place their trust in the Internet as a means to motivate commerce will affect consumers' intentions to return to a web site. Competence trust has a significant influence on consumers' pre- and postpurchase decisions. Further, competence trust affects consumer satisfaction. Consumers, however, are concerned about doing business on-line.

Some 65% of on-line customers bail out of a transaction before the final step. Information satisfaction then becomes a critical component to consider in the design of a web site, there must be a strategy that supports repeat customers.

SIGNIFICANCE OF ELECTRONIC COMMERCE

Electronic commerce has led to dramatic changes in the definition of a firm. From electronic commerce over the Internet has emerged virtual companies that are capable of delivering products and services largely because they are able to create and maintain a network of business relationships. The three significant benefits of using electronic commerce are:

- — Reducing cost for routine business transactions;
- — Collapsing cycle time to complete business transactions, regardless of geographic dispersion; and
- — Eliminating paper and inefficiencies in handling paper.

Four business benefit criteria to evaluate the potential for electronic markets, including:

- — Extending the firm's reach.
- — Bypassing traditional channels.

— Augmenting traditional markets.

— Boosting service and advertising.

Extending the firm's reach refers to the firm's ability to reach any potential customer, regardless of geographic location. Bypassing traditional channels refers to the ability to reduce dependence upon intermediaries. Augmenting traditional markets refers to the emergence of new means for marketing products and services. Boosting service refers to the ability to utilize electronic commerce 24 hours per day.

Advertising assumes special significance in an electronic commerce market. Firms are not constrained by boundaries of length, time, and place. A model of electronic commerce consisting of three elements: content, context, and infrastructure. In the electronic marketplace, content is information-based, with a focus on electronic transactions. The context of marketing via electronic commerce changes from a real to a virtual environment that is available any time, any place.

The infrastructure, where transactions occur, is completely different as well. Electronic commerce changes the context of product and place in its definitional context. The use of the Internet as a channel of distribution enables interactive commerce to occur. The term interactive as consisting of two features of communication: the ability to address an individual and the ability to gather and remember that individual's response.

When a consumer visits a web site, many exchange cycles can occur within a brief time period. Moreover, when a consumer returns to a web site, exchanges can resume where the previous exchange left off. In addition to time independence, one benefit to consumers is that they need not repeat previously-entered information to resume interrupted transactions. Marketing on the web dilutes the difference between large and small companies, enabling them to perform one-on-one marketing.

One-on-one marketing as the ability to use information about an individual to market specific products or services that are assumed to be of interest to that individual. While this is not a new concept, the use of the Internet has opened a new channel of distribution, based on the premise that if a company can develop a personal relationship with a consumer, the consumer will continue to buy more products or services from that company.

Two categories of data as essential for enabling one-on-one marketing. The first is the variety of needs an individual consumer is looking to satisfy through the firm's products or services. The second is the value skew of the distribution of profits that current customers generate for the firm. Dividing the variety and value presents a customer differentiation matrix. This matrix of low to high value and skewness can help define the electronic commerce strategy for the firm.

One useful outcome of this approach is that a company can learn from the data it collects. If a company begins with the wrong electronic commerce strategy but effectively monitors and controls its web site, it can more easily make interim adjustments until it achieves the right mix of differentiation.

It was necessary to examine the user's overlapping roles and technical perspectives to create an effective e-commerce strategy. Several areas must be evaluated to understand the effect of consumer response from ecommerce. The first is web site design. Various factors affect web site design, the most important factor being page-loading speed. Consumers who do business electronically do not want to wait while web pages are downloaded.

The use of graphics, animated gifs, and files that require plug – in device drivers to maximise page – loading speed. Additionally, the use of plugins should be avoided because the average person does not want to download and install software in order to return and access a web site successfully. Nor should graphics be overlooked as an important way to distinguish between web sites. To effectively compete in an electronic commerce environment, a company's e-commerce strategy should address, among other issues, how it will handle graphics.

One way is through the use of thumbnails, which can be expanded into larger pictures. With myriad options available to consumers who are doing business electronically, an effective web site strategy will consider the transmission speed that a consumer is likely to utilize and design appropriately. The business content of the web site should contain clear concise language that readily describes the business. It should also include contact information via telephone and/or email for user follow-up. The web site content should be changed regularly to remain attractive for repeat customers.

Navigation efficiency refers to the easy use of the entire set of web pages. A well-defined web site should have no broken or non-existing links. The use of frames garnered mixed responses. On the plus side, they break up the web page, provide more flexible functionality, and display the company logo across each page. Among the disadvantages are that frames are not supported by older browsers and make bookmarking more difficult. Frames can also add horizontal and vertical scrolling to a page.

Whether or not frames are used, however, navigation should be consistent throughout a well-defined web site. An e-commerce strategy should also define other factors that affect web site design. These factors include the business content of the web site, navigation, efficiency, security, and customer focus. It is important to consider the existing telecommunications infrastructure when defining an e-commerce strategy. Because it is consumed at a rapid rate, telecommunications bandwidth should be considered when designing resource intensive web sites.

Marketing to businesses that utilize T1 lines to access a company's web site may present different design options than marketing to consumers who access the web site via a 28.8 or 56.6 modem. More than 75% of Internet traffic is HTTP-related. Network planning is critical to obtaining acceptable user response time. It is important to consider what type of web server an organisation needs to compete in an electronic commerce market.

There is no one single type of web server. Web servers can be used as proxy servers, electronic commerce servers, or search engines that are image-intensive and highly dynamic or primarily static. E-commerce consists of two domains: business-to-business inter-organisation systems, usually implemented via electronic data interchange (EDI), and electronic markets that exist on the World Wide Web.

The World Wide Web has been described as having two primary roles. First, it serves as a distribution channel that allows the quick delivery of products and services via the Internet. A consumer can not only order goods, but also obtain an on-line view of exactly how they will look prior to delivery.

Service models are used in an e-commerce environment to support customers or provide additional products or services. The types of services identified were: product/service updates, inquiry processes, frequently asked questions (FAQs), and transaction tracking. A good example of transaction tracking can be found on the United States Postal Service website. For an additional charge, a customer can receive a number with which to track the status of a mailed item. Exchange models are used to offer products or services for sale.

The types of exchanges identified were on-line catalogs, targeted marketing, integrated sales, and integrated sales fulfillment. Targeted marketing seeks to influence customer behaviour through customer profiles, customised information, and narrow cast messages. Integrated sales link front-end and back-end sales activities through the web site. For example, Dell Corporation has effectively integrated its entire sales operation through the Web and dramatically reduced its cost structure by integrating its operation with its supporting vendors.

Dell automatically triggers UPS at three different times to pick up a PC, monitor, and software to synchronise their arrival at a customer's location. This integrated marketing strategy distinguishes effective e-commerce marketing and will become more widely used as companies expand into the e-commerce marketplace. Web site performance management needs to be integrated into an e-commerce strategy.

Firms with clearly-defined web objectives have firmer performance measures to evaluate the actual performance of their web site than firms without defined web site objectives. Further research to measure the linkage between web site performance and achieving the firm's business objectives. Specific metrics can determine if the web site is achieving these objectives. Special performance considerations, such as web pre-fetching, may be needed.

Web pre-fetching is a strategy of loading documents into a client's web site before the user has selected them for browsing, thus reducing the user's access time. Pre-fetching can be characterised as client-side or server-side, depending upon which device initiated the prefetch operation. The longer the estimated time to retrieve web pages, the more likely they will be pre-fetched. Web pages that are quick to fetch, dynamically generated or beyond certain limits will not be pre-fetched.

EFFECTIVE WEB SITE DESIGN

Effective web site design can be more rapidly developed utilizing prototyping, which is useful for developing a proof of concept to quickly determine the web site's cost effectiveness. Four steps in web site prototyping.

The first step, define needs, involves identifying and articulating the client's description of what the users want. The second step, define ideas, extracts concepts from all of the participants and turns them into a meaningful entity. Step three, design, builds an entity that is the culmination of all ideas. The final step, deliver, is bringing specifications to the client to construct the application. This is based upon the assumption that once the prototype is developed (as part of the design step), the client will be responsible to transform it into a production-ready application.

This can be useful in determining the cost benefits of web site development and support. The rapid surge of electronic commerce has allowed existing industries, such as telecommunications providers, to expand their support services. As well, new industries, such as infomediaries, are better able to help consumers find businesses on-line for their own growth.

New markets and increased electronic commerce have resulted in businesses transforming themselves to remain competitive. Full cyber-marketing organisations that operate exclusively through the Internet have emerged rapidly. A well-designed web site should result in developing a customer base that will more likely purchase goods and services on-line. Customers are expected to purchase more because of the complete, timely, and effective presentation of web site information.

Two significant marketing factors that affect electronic commerce. Time-specific assets have value if they reach users within a specified time period. The complexity of the product description determines the amount of detail information that a consumer needs to make a purchase decision. Together, these lead to the electronic integration effect, which occurs when information technology is used not only to speed communication but to change the processes that create and use information. The use of the Internet as a channel for electronic commerce capitalises on these factors.

INFLUENCE WEB RELATIONSHIP – BUILDING

Loyalty and Trust

Loyalty programmes are being introduced to e-commerce marketing as a way to build relationships with customers. Affective and conative loyalty can influence customers' perceptions of products. Affective loyalty, for example, may influence how well customers speak about a product. Conative loyalty, on the other hand, may determine whether customers continue to buy products into the future.

European banks on what determines loyalty when bank services move from the traditional marketplace to on-line commerce. They found that customer satisfaction, followed by brand reputation, had the greatest impact on both affective and conative customer loyalty. Two other determinants in the study, switching costs and search costs, had less influence on loyalty.

Readers of The Wall Street Journal typically have a strong loyalty to the printed version of the newspaper.

Yet when customers buy an electronic version of it, they expect that the reading experience will match that of the printed version in delivering high-quality business news. The electronic version, of course, has a potential for greater success if customers remain satisfied and loyal. Organisations that choose to build a web relationship with their customers find it an effective way of developing brand loyalty.

Manufacturers and retailers are also learning that treating their customers as faceless individuals jeopardises their loyalty and future business. Four loyalty drivers that influence customer buying decisions, which also apply to web sites and web entities:

— Product offering,

— Quality,

— Price, and

— Image.

Most organisations understand the power of the first three-product, quality, and price. The image driver or relationship-building driver, however, determines whether an organisation retains its loyal customers for the future. Companies need to work at creating e-loyalty. "What the web does for e-loyalty is make building relationships easier, faster, and cheaper". People who are loyal to each other can also be loyal to web sites.

Another strategy for building e-loyalty for a web site is intelligent dialogue, implying that Web interactions must sound, feel, and appear human to create successful relationships. Extending beyond merely providing web information such as flights on line, for example, the site must offer customers real – time valuable information about flight cancellations, ways to rebook, and a toll – free number for advice. In addition, this information must be delivered in a timely format attractive to the customers. The nature of intelligent dialogue is influenced by the type of product offered, the customer's sex, education, and age, and the culture of the organisation. It will also be based on research of customer values that influence buying decisions.

The rationale for making e-loyalty work as a strategy on the web is based upon sound business principles:

- Retaining customers is more costeffective than acquiring new ones;
- Loyal customers are typically more profitable as a segment based on lifetime purchasing value than non-loyal customers;
- Loyal customers defect less often; and
- Loyal customers are more likely to boost one's brand and image.

In sum, on-line customer loyalty can only be achieved with a close bond between seller and buyer. As active participants in the transaction, customers will often recommend the organisation to friends, family, and co-workers.

Community Building On-line

Just as the Industrial Revolution prompted people from their communities to find work and share interests with others, virtual communities are becoming the social organising mechanism to unite consumers in the 21st century. Because customers apparently want to meet and share information in cyberspace, this development has triggered the need to expand on-line communities among members with common interests. This power of community-building is not lost on information technology and public relations executives who are challenged by trying to satisfy customers on-line.

The Web is slowly becoming America's collective "town square," a place to buy products, find medical advice, join a club or self-help group, play games, trade items, and share information and news through e-mail and chat rooms. As part of an on-line community, customers are no longer limited to joining local neighborhood groups or buying locally; their reach has become national and global, while also choosing to remain anonymous or declare their identity on-line.

Community-building on the web is a relatively new public relations strategy which gained momentum once the Internet was launched and became a community of dialogue. For example, a company's communication on the Web can elicit immediate response from customers, creating a wave of positive or negative publicity that directly impacts the organisation's image. Four categories of on-line communities: geography, demographics, topic, and shared activities.

These categories provide a typology for sharing information and ascertaining and meeting customers' common needs. It is important to note that on-line communities are not static and should evolve over time; Village, for example, renamed itself the Women's Network after it discovered that its members were interested in parenting, health, relationships, and money issues.

Communities on the Web have humanised the on-line experience by letting individuals use message boards that provide a live link or a feeling of personal involvement with the organisation. Real-time chatting is another form of customer interaction. New software for real-time chatting allows for synchronous communication among residents in different parts of the world. Companies can also schedule special on-line events for their customers, thus attracting a crowd of compatible consumers to their web site.

Furthermore, to build strong relationships with customers on the Web, companies should offer real-time support and guidance. A live support option is a good complement to FAQs (frequently asked questions) because it can increase the probability that customers will return to the site to purchase more products or services. One of the best ways to ensure success on the Web is to understand the qualities that a community values the most.

In the auto sector, for example, price, design, and service are important, while in the fashion industry, style, brand, and freedom of choice are drivers that influence buying habits. Effective public relations strategies allow the organisation to express these qualities through web design, image, language, and feedback. To stand out from the competition, organisations must communicate a distinctive persona. In the final analysis, e-marketers need to understand that content alone may lure visitors to a site initially, but their decision to stay is tied in with discovering a community that shares their values.

For example, the community aspects of the Women's Network define its shared values. Its "better health" section resembles a visit to a local spa with experts offering healthrelated advice. Whether an auto company promotes a fan club for its most famous car brands or movie stars contact their on-line fan clubs around the world, the power of community shapes both image and brand, and humanises the Web's digital experience.

e-COMMERCE WEB SITE DESIGN MODEL

The e-commerce web site design model (Figure 1) provides a framework to explain the type of marketing and public relations integration needed to support consumer satisfaction. The model assumes that consumers in a B2C (business-to-consumer) environment access web sites either because:

— They seek information about a specific product or service;

— They require specific choices about products or services, including complimentary or substitute products; or

— They seek to make on-line purchases.

Electronic commerce web sites attempt to satisfy consumers' needs through one of four classifications of integrated marketing-technological strategy. These four classifications-introductory, informative, interactive, intelligence-explain how an organisation chooses to organise and present its web site as well as what consumers desire and how they will respond.

Organisations seek to optimize responses to the desired goal of the web site when they have an effective integrated marketing plan. Each classification represents a specific set of design characteristics for web sites (Table 1). Each web site classification should have a public relations dimension to build customer loyalty and enhance the probability that the customer will frequently return to the site to buy products.

Every customer interaction is an opportunity to make a sale or make a friend. The public relations dimension can build support for a site in three important ways: credibility, cachet, and community. Credibility is a value-added process because it generates an audience's willingness to believe that the business will be sucessful.

Table 1: Web Site Classification

Web Site Classification	Desired Response Definitional Criteria
Introductory	Firms in this category establish a web site identify their products and services.
Informative	Firms in this category use their web site to direct customers to specific locations,

	including other web sites, in order to complete transactions purchases.
Interactive	Firms in this category design web sites that interact with consumers, primarily in the form of transaction processing. Consumers are given immediate feedback once a purchase transaction has been completed.
Intelligence	Firms in this category utilize intelligent agents to build and maintain customer profiles. Web sites are personalised to respond to individual consumer needs.

A special feeling from the site that intrigues consumers enough to return to it. Key influencers can drive traffic to a site with a mere mention in a major magazine, national newspaper or network.

Finally, community consists of online customers who dialogue with the organisation through e-mail or other feedback mechanisms and share their interests and concerns about the organisation's products or services. For example, Sony and Yahoo have strong public relations dimensions on their sites that help build customer trust and loyalty.

PUBLIC RELATIONS STRATEGY DIMENSION

The introductory site might have a distinctive logo, a tailored message from the CEO, an annual report or press releases to help build good will and customer loyalty. The informative site may choose to use testimonials from satisfied customers or celebrities who have used the products or services.

The interactive site may include a video message from the CEO or a video that shows how the transaction is completed and the product will be delivered. A pledge or endorsement similar to the Good Housekeeping Seal of Approval may be used to build credibility or trust.

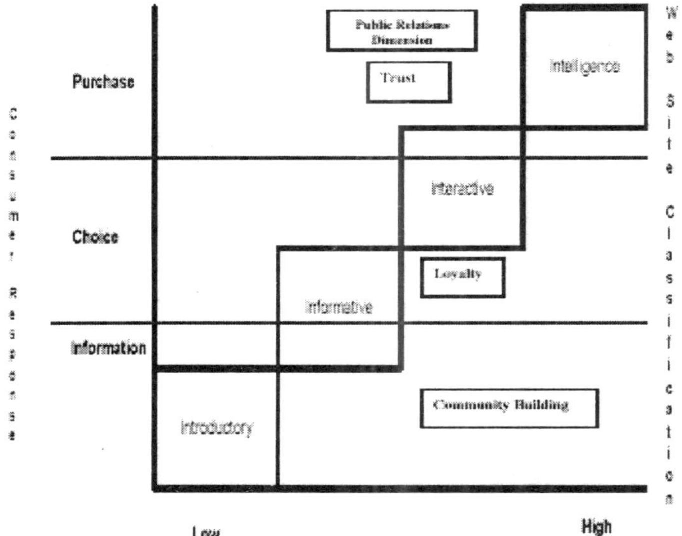

Figure 1: Model of E-Commerce Web Site Design

It also includes ways to humanise the digital experience and build strong communities that share common experiences.

Organisation: Dependence on e-commerce

The intelligence site has options for personal customer feedback and opinions, including a money-back guarantee with the option to talk with a representative on an 800 number if necessary to close the sale. Community dialogue options and cachet are for important to lure customers back to this site. Organisations competing in the world of e-commerce must develop e-commerce strategies to guide and maintain their web site development.

These strategies should define which type of e-commerce web site classification the organisations employ and they should be updated as organisational needs change. Organisations that rely heavily on e-commerce will more likely utilize interactive and intelligence-based web site designs. The ecommerce web site design model postulates the following:

— *P1:* Consumer response is affected by web site design.

— *P2:* An organisation's web site design is affected by its dependence upon e-commerce as a channel of distribution.

— *P3:* Consumer satisfaction increases when the web site design classification matches the desired response.

Consumer satisfaction is an important determinant in evaluating electronic commerce as a long-term strategic technology that benefits and enhances the firm. As part of that strategy, a well-designed public relations dimension would enrich customer satisfaction and loyalty. By integrating public relations into web site design, organisations can strengthen their relationships on the web; build brand awareness that promotes loyalty in their customers' hearts and minds; and create on-line communities that share values with the company.

Today, a strong Web presence is becoming more imperative than traditional marketing communications tools such as fancy brochures, direct mail, and select advertising. The e-commerce web site design model provides a framework for analysing how a web site design with a public relations dimension impacts consumer satisfaction.

Further empirical testing is planned to validate the relationship between web site design classification and consumer satisfaction. Additionally, a sampling of web sites will be conducted to support the web site classifications. In particular, one method will sample web sites by industry type to assess the significance of industry type. Data mining on the Web is an emerging technology.

Companies highly dependent on electronic commerce and utilizing intelligence-based web sites are interested in evaluating consumers' purchasing and browsing patterns. Future work will focus on evaluating consumer satisfaction through data-mining as a means of creating intelligence-based web sites as well as on public relation strategies that support data mining-based web sites. Imagery impacts consumer intention to return to a web site, this future work will consider image mining in addition to text mining.

The most important attributes of measuring good relationships are trust, understanding, credibility, behaviour, mutuality of control or conflict avoidance, and maintenance of that existing relationship between an organisation and its key constituencies. If organisations are serious about understanding the type of experience their customers are having on their web site, they should employ qualitative and quantitative gathering techniques such as exploratory customer focus groups, representative mail and telephone surveys of current and lapsed customers, and in-depth interviews on customer buying habits.

Qualitative focus groups can also be utilized with on-line user groups to learn which values and buying habits customers consider important. Quantitative mail and telephone surveys should follow to confirm statistically the findings of the focus groups. An easy method for keeping track of customers' opinions and behaviours on the Web is through feedback loops, both conversational and behavioural.

Conversational feedback includes e-mail, message boards, chat sessions, and interviews, while behavioural feedback includes page hits, time spent on site, message boards and chat sessions, and responses to direct marketing. Feedback loops provide excellent clues to how effectively a web site offering matches the needs and values of its key constituencies. Additional ways that organisations can learn about their e-commerce relationships with customers. First, customer advisory panels for B2B customers are useful, particularly if organisations are trying to build long-term relationships.

Second, employee surveys measure how well organisations are delivering quality service on the Web. Finally, mystery shoppers can be used to test the Web site experience by buying a product and reporting their experiences. Finally, Microsoft's Usability Guidelines (MUG) can be a valuable metric to assess the quality of a firm's Web presence. These guidelines are organised into five major categories:

— Content,

— Ease of use,

— Promotion,

— Made for the medium (personalisation), and

— Emotion (affective).

A heuristic evaluation procedure using multiple web sites from four sectors engaged in electronic commerce: airlines, on-line bookstores, automobile manufacturers, and car rental agencies. They noted that the evaluation procedure as well as the usability metric exhibited good properties. Three of the categories-promotion, made for the medium, and emotion-have public relations aspects directly related to building relationships that support customer satisfaction.

9

USING INTERNET FOR COMMUNITY INFORMATION

Internet use has the reverse effect by isolating individuals and decreasing interpersonal interaction. Despite the lauding of the internet's potential for strengthening physical communities by facilitating information flow about local resources and civic interaction through formal and informal channels. Life in an electronic world poses several fundamental problems. Equitable and easy access to information about local resources can help people deal with the myriad situations that arise through everyday living such as finding a new job, locating daycare services, dealing with grief or divorce, moving to a new neighborhood, finding where to get your car fixed, etc.

All people – despite their education, financial status, occupation, or social ties – experience situations where they have difficulties in recognising, expressing, and meeting their needs for such community information (CI). Barriers including cultural, financial, geographic, and physical further challenge users with successfully seeking CI such that they cannot always obtain information about needed services or participate fully in civic life.

Although information technologies hold significant promise for linking individuals with information and one another, they are foreshadowed by the potential for a deeper digital divide between the information rich and the information poor. Recognising the importance of CI for making a difference in people's lives and, on a related level, for creating and sustaining healthy communities, many public libraries have focused on providing three types of CI: human services information, local information, and citizen action information.

In addition to providing CI through information and referral (I&R) services since the 1970s, public libraries organised and supported communitywide information initiatives with local service providers. The internet, however, along with faster connectivity, wider variety of enabled devices, and enhanced graphical user interfaces, has suggested new ways for libraries to facilitate the publicz's everyday information needs through digital CI systems.

One such digital collaboration in which libraries have played a leading role since the 1980s, and which is flourishing worldwide, is community networking. These networks provide the public with one-stop shopping using community-oriented discussions, question-and-answer forums, access to governmental and social services, along with local information, email, and internet access.

Although individuals may interact with other users by posting queries, monitoring discussions, etc., CI is often a central network feature that appears in many forms: libraries, for example, may make their databases accessible through the internet, while individual social service and other providers can post information about their programmes. Thus, the architecture of the internet makes digital CI possible by linking information files created not only by single organisations such as libraries, but by agencies, organisations, and individuals throughout the community.

This is a major departure from traditional I&R services where librarians and other CI agency staff work with files about the community that are created on an internal library system. As a result of digital CI systems accessible through community networks, people can access CI through public library terminals-or any internet-enabled device regardless of location-while seeking help with related information search techniques from librarians. In short, digital systems mean that citizens can access CI anytime, in any place.

To date, little is known about how access to digital CI systems help (or do not help) citizens with daily living, how CI affects their information behavior, and how it may or may not benefit communities. It was observed that research interest in citizens' use of networked CI is increasing. However, the majority of artricles reviewed were applied and descriptive in nature, and based on questionnaires or analysed transaction log data that focused on user socio-demographics and system or access statistics such as page use frequency.

Most studies were from the professional literature and reported conflicting user and use statistics. In this sense, the networked CI system literature has been akin to the general public library literature that Zweizig and Dervin criticised as providing little insight into the uses that people make of information and information systems.

Through interviews and focus groups in low-income neighborhoods with users and potential users of the Prairienet community network, they identified the following categories of digital CI need: community services and activities, resources for children, healthcare, education, employment, crime and safety, and general reference tools. Librarians might provide more effective digital information services if they focus on ways that complement citizens' lifestyles, constraints, and information seeking patterns.

ELECTRONIC WORLD

In this chapter we are discussing about the findings from a recent study of how public libraries are using on-line community networks to facilitate the public's information seeking and use in everyday situations, conducted in United States. The study team used multiple methods to collect data over several stages. Stage one of the study consisted of a survey with 500 medium and large-sized public libraries regarding their involvement with digital CI systems. For stage two, the study team used a standard case study design to conduct intensive research in three communities that received had national recognition for their respective community network and in which the local public library system played a leading role.

Both the on-line user survey and follow-up interviews were based on Dervin's sense-making methodology, which comprises a set of user-centered assumptions and methods for studying the uses individuals make of information systems. It asserts that throughout daily life, people encounter gaps in their knowledge that they can only fill or bridge by making new sense of their situations through seeking information. Thus, they use varied strategies to seek and construct information from different resources or ideas as they cope with different barriers, which Dervin and Frenette explain using the sense-making metaphor (Fig. 1). Sense-making facilitates the study of different aspects of information behavior.

The study included two dimensions:

(a) users' assessments of the helpfulness of digital CI, and

(b) users' and service providers' constructions or images of these systems.

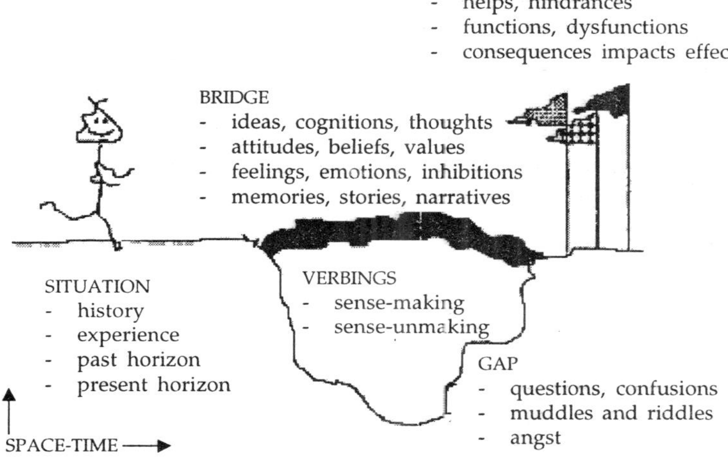

Figure 1: Sense-making metaphor

Both were investigated using Dervin's micro-moment time-line technique where respondents were asked "to reconstruct a situation in terms of what happe-ned (time-line steps) and then to describe each step in detail". This enabled the study team to gather and comp-are perceptions of different players regarding how CI is constructed and used through electronic communication.

Use of Networked CI Systems

The age of the 197 individuals who responded to the online survey followed a normal distribution with most respondents (71.4%) falling between the ages of 25 and 55, and slightly more women (54.6%) responded than men. The findings of the study suggest that a typical user is nonexistent, socio-demographically speaking: users equally represent men and women, a distributed range of age groups, and a diverse range of occupations: from students to blue-collar workers to white-collar professionals.

Networked CI systems were used by the respondents for many different types of situations, including work-related and those of a personal nature. This confirms a tenet of information behavior, namely that all individuals require CI at one point or another and that it is the individual's situation that provides the greater insight into information seeking and use. Users seek the following types of digital CI:

— Business
— Computer/technical
— Education
— Employment
— Financial support
— Governmental/civic
— Health
— Housing
— Library operations and services
— Local events
— Local history and genealogy
— Local information
— Local news
— Organisations and groups
— Other people
— Parenting
— Recreation and hobbies
— Sale, exchange, or donation of goods
— Social services
— Volunteerism

Examples of how respondents used the community networks included:

(a) teenagers who sought summer employment information because they believed the community network contained all the local job information in one place and trusted it as a reliable, current source;

(b) a man who found a local directory of gay and lesbian organisations on his commuity network after finding only national resources on the Web;

(c) a home-bound person who used the network to research his family's genealogy because of its comprehensive organisation of local resources, including public library, county agency and local historical association materials; and,

(d) a woman who used the network for such local government information as current ordinances pertaining to trash pickup and flood damage prevention, and to identify sources of funding for a community service project intended to help a nearby low-income community.

The above CI categories expand upon those reported by Bisho, et al. and are markedly broader than those traditionally used to classify CI. Chen and Hernon, for example, classified their data using seven categories (consumer issues, housing, education, recreation, health, personal relations, and other). The study put a strong emphasis on employment opportunities, volunteerism, social service availability, local history and genealogy, It included new categories such as: sale, exchange and donation of goods, local news, computer and technical information, and other people.

According to sense-making theory, information needs cannot be considered in isolation of the situations in which they emerged, because any situation is likely to yield multiple information needs: information found for one aspect of a query frequently opens another, related information need. The situations for which users sought digital CI were complex and usually required multiple pieces of information. This notion of the ongoing search is similar to Bates' "berrypicking" concept where users search for information "a bit at a time" and alter their search strategies according to what they find and what barriers they encounter.

In analysing the CI that users sought by need category, the study also focused on the information's enabling aspects, i.e., the attributes of the information that would aid users in whatever it was they were trying to accomplish. Nine information "enabling" characteristics for classifying the types of CI requested by citizens and nonprofit organisation leadership. These enabling attributes provide an extended way of viewing information needs because they focus on what users are trying to accomplish for a particular situation and why they were helped by seeking a particular type of CI. When considered in conjunction with (a) the user's initial need, (b) the situation that prompted that need, and (c) what is known about the barriers that users encounter-as discussed next-these enabling categories reveal several implications for the design of digital CI systems.

Barriers to Using CI Systems

Barriers, a key concept in the sense-making framework, represent the ways in which people are prevented or blocked from seeking information-or, more broadly, getting help-successfully. By identifying barriers, one can devise ways of improving the design of digital CI systems that facilitate users' information seeking.

Several open-ended questions that addressed types of barriers. Specifically, if anything, would make it easier for them to find what they're looking for, and to describe any past actions they might have taken regarding their search topic. Despite respondents' confidence in their abilities to get higher quality information, they encountered a range of barriers to access along the way.

Several basic types of barriers to using community networks and the internet, in general. These barriers were: technological (e.g., slow connection speeds and software, unavailable or incompatible systems), economic (e.g., users could not afford computing equipment or online access), geographic, search skills (users did not know how to search the system/internet or how to use advanced methods), cognitive (users did not understand how the internet works in terms of how links are created, who creates and manages the information, how sites are updated, etc.), and psychological (users expressed a lack of confidence in their own ability to find needed information, i.e., they internalised search failures and believed the reason they could not find something was because they were unable to carry out the search successfully).

In addition to these basic barrier types, the main barrier that identified in the study was information related. It encompassed several subcategories:

- *Poor Retrieval-Information Overload and Low Precision*: Due to poor search engines and site indexing, users retrieved too much CI and were challenged with discerning what was relevant to their search;
- *Poor Interface Design*: Users were often daunted by a site's layout (appeared too busy, too many bells and whistles, poor font and color choice, especially for those who are color-blind) and the amount of text displayed on a single screen;
- *Poorly Organised (Classified)*: Users did not find CI where they expected to find it, and there was little crossreferencing;

— *Out-of-Date and Inaccurate Information*: CI was either out of date or there was no way of discerning when a page was created or last updated. Inaccuracies in content were also noted;

— *Authority*: Without proper identifiers and author credentials or association endorsements, users found it difficult to gauge the quality of the CI source, i.e., whether they should trust the CI (and its source) or not;

— *Missing*: Users sometimes commented that information was missing, although it was described as existing at the beginning of a page or document;

— *Dead Links*: Users were frustrated when finding a link to a page or site that they believe would be highly relevant to their information need, only to find that the link was inactive or otherwise unavailable;

— *Language Used*: Beyond most information appearing in English only, some sites contained information written in jargon or at a level too high to understand;

— *Security*: Users want strong evidence that the information they submit and retrieve is confidential;

— *Specificity*: Users wanted to search for information at the neighborhood level and to find people;

— *Nonanticipatory Systems*: Uses indicated that their information behavior would be greatly facilitated if CI systems were smart enough either to anticipate their next information need or a related information need. All too often users described how the site they found was not quite what they were looking for but they did not know where to go to next.

In addition to the barriers noted earlier, these information-related barriers are highly significant because they represent specific impediments that users encounter when seeking information. Job seekers, for example, feel that they cannot get ahead unless they have access to a computer, not only so they can become more computer literate, but also because that's how they perceive that people learn about job opportunities these days.

For any one situation or information need, a user might be confronted by several barriers, which, collectively, can overwhelm the user and prevent him or her from locating needed information. These barriers point to problems as well as potential solutions for improving the usability and helpfulness of digital CI systems. Despite these information-related barriers, some respondents were highly confident that they could find what they needed through the community network. They tended to perceive their community network as a ubiquitous source and gateway to all knowledge. In this sense the study team identified a mismatch between what users think they can obtain via the internet and the likelihood that that information exists and can be easily located. This finding expands on a principle of everyday information behavior: that a mismatch exists between what users believe service providers offer and what they actually do.

PUBLIC'S ONLINE INFORMATION BEHAVIOR

Since the 1960s, information science research has indicated that social ties and face-to-face communication are primary sources of information, regardless of the setting. The internet has not replaced the role of social ties in citizens' information behavior. During the interviews, several respondents described how they spoke about their information need or situation with a social tie before searching on-line.

Thus, he internet is supplementing other information seeking behaviors in addition to creating new pathways for obtaining information: the public is using digital CI systems as an additional source, which supports a key finding from pre-internet studies: that people employ multiple sources based on such factors as accessibility and ease of use. Moreover, the study found that people want their community networks to promote social interaction by bringing people together. This notion was expressed by a user who said: "a bulletin board or some way to facilitate people meeting each other and getting around would be very helpful. I've recently moved to town and am looking for ways to meet people. Maybe a place where people could find others who are interested in a supper club or playing cards, or informal sporting groups, etc."

This notion that users want the internet to help them increase social ties and social capital is supported by Wellman, Haase, Witte, and Hampton, who reported that communicating on-line is supplementing face-to-face and telephone communication, and that heavy internet use is associated with increased participation in voluntary organisations and politics. Further evidence that the internet may foster social cohesion came from respondents, who revealed that they were searching for CI on behalf of another person, and not always at that person's behest.

The internet has made it easier for researchers to label and identify a particular social type, one that might be best described as "information gatherers" or "monitors" to borrow from Baker and Pettigrew. These active CI seekers, who may be considered similar to information gatekeepers, relished time spent browsing and poking about the community network and the internet. But their greatest satisfaction was when they found something that they believed might be of interest to someone else, which they would quickly pass on, either by e-mail or in person.

Hence, a distinguishing feature of these CI gatherers is that they are socially connected or active, and, perhaps more importantly, are aware of the potential CI needs or interests of people they know. They take mental notes of what's going on in the lives of the people around them, their interests and situations, and then keep an eye out for CI that might be of interest or helpful-not by initiating an actual, purposive search. In this sense, they are able to recognise the potential CI needs of the people around them and match it with available online information.

Another defining element of this social type is that they do not really care if the CI they pass on is actually used, and they exhibit an understanding that sometimes information is used and proven helpful at a later point in time. This information gatherer social type has implications for systems design.

In communities, for example, that are considered information poor, individuals who represent this social type could be identified and given advance training in internet searching as well as in how to identify information needs and how to provide information in ways that best facilitate those needs. Respondents used the community network as a personal gateway to Web sites located throughout the world, while people far beyond the network's physical home were using it to obtain local information.

Individuals and Builds Community

Despite the barriers that users encounter when seeking community information on-line, the participants in the study overwhelming emphasised how they have benefited from the availability of on-line CI via their community networks. An increased ability to access community information. Specifically, they described how they now have:

— Increased access to hard to get information;

— Increased access to "higher quality" information (i.e., more current, more comprehensive, better organised, and linked to other relevant sites);

— Information that is easier to use;

— Decreased transaction "costs" (saving them time, money, and energy; increased convenience); and,

— Increased ability to identify trusted information.

Users also described how access to networked community information yielded benefits at the personal, family, and neighborhood levels. Specifically, they described how community networks have provided them with:

— Greater confidentiality protection and greater comfort in asking sensitive questions;

— Greater skill and confidence building;

— Employment and educational gains;

— Increased knowledge of community; and,

— Value for family, friends, and neighborhood.

Support for these themes emerged repeatedly. People explained how their local community network provided them with one-stop shopping for information about all aspects of their area and met the information needs of their entire families. One user commented on how relocating to the city was made easier by the network.

Both users and other stakeholders, including social service and public library staff, reported benefiting from the ways in which public library-community network initiatives build community and facilitate cohesiveness both within and among different subpopulations. Leaders of community nonprofit organisations, specifically, elucidated upon how they have received the following benefits as a result of participating in their local community network:

- More effective at service provision;
- Enhanced visibility-word gets out to more folks, wider audience, additional, volunteers and support;
- More tuned into the internet and its benefits;
- Knowledge/skill and confidence building;
- Information technology helps them better serve community; and,
- Decreased transaction costs.

Sense-Making

Model of the sense-making methodology to map teh study findings regarding users' on-line information behavior. Sense-making contains several main concepts: the user's situation that creates his/her needs for information, the barriers that the user encounters in expressing those needs and while seeking information, and the results or "helps" that the user obtained through the course of successfully information seeking. Collectively, the analysis of users' information behavior and the benefits accrued by users and other stakeholders suggests that on-line community networks are transforming physical communities into information communities. In other words, the internet has facilitated the creation of information communities-an emerging concept that describes constituencies united by a common interest in building and increasing access to a set of dynamic, linked, and varying information resources.

Common foundations and shared principles offset the uniqueness of different information communities. They are, for example, likely to be dynamic and distributed (in technological terms), and involve the collaboration of a variety of organisations that may share joint responsibility and resources (including in-kind contributions). Moreover, information communities form around people's needs to get and use information-concepts of which their leaders have some understanding.

Because these communities effectively exploit the information-sharing qualities of the internet, they tend to incorporate diverse information providers, use collaborative approaches, communicate across geographic and other barriers, and adopt entrepreneurial approaches. Although some information communities are based on geographic boundaries, others are based on thematic interests.

10

PUBLIC RELATIONS ETHICS

Any effective unit in teaching should begin with a definition of terms-even when the term is as complex as ethics. This gives you and your students a common starting point. Students find it helpful to begin with a simple, easily-grasped definition. It is helpful, also, to distinguish between law and ethics. Law can be thought of as a body of actions mandated by society. It establishes the minimum rules of conduct to which everyone who lives in that society is obligated to adhere, and it covers a wide range of behavior, from murder to speed limits.

Ethics are concerned with what people should do as opposed to what we are obliged to do. They incorporate a variety of values-societal, religious, cultural, etc.- and provide a basis for making decisions about actions. Ethics are voluntary-they are a system for making decisions when no rule or law exists to mandate behavior. Ethics are values in action.

Values are socially constructed—we, as a people, develop some sort of consensus as to what is of importance. Religion is frequently noted as a major force in the shaping of values in a society, but religion is itself a social construction that has been institutionalised. Values change over time: they are a product of and contributor to the political, economic, social and cultural environment of the society in which they are practiced. Behrman, for example, cites the following as some of the key values in our society today: honesty, status, equity, stewardship, charity, justice, efficiency, love, reverence, diligence, progress, truth, loyalty, brotherhood, mercy, cleanliness, orderliness, prudence. This understanding of values results in an understanding of ethics, which are based on values, as being situated in time and space.

Understanding of values becomes extremely important when exploring historical and international situations. Melvin Sharpe illustrates this nicely: Global interdependence, new technology, population growth and knowledge advancements are now confronting human society continually with new ethical questions. As global society learns new causes of cancer and other illnesses, results of pollution and environmental destruction and the social consequences of certain products and actions, new ethical values emerge that were unheeded and in some cases unneeded in previous periods of time.

The present social ability to analyse social consequences and to communicate the analysis beyond the ability of previous generations lets us look, evaluate, debate and formulate entirely new social norms. Previously acceptable individual and organisational social behavior can be labeled unacceptable more rapidly than in any previous time period simply due to advancements in communication technology.

Public relations itself is a hybrid that has spent most of this century evolving into its own unique and discrete breed, its ethical roots are entangled with those of its predecessors: business and journalism. If we say a practitioner should be ethical; and if we acknowledge that some professional organisations, like the Public Relations Society of America, police their members to make sure they are acting in accord with the profession's code of ethics, then the question to be answered becomes:

How does a professional make ethical decisions? Many decisions people make-as individuals and as professionals-fall in the domain of ethics. Therefore, students need a system for making good decisions. One way to approach ethics is to look at them in terms of "isms:" utilitarianism, absolutism, rationalism, situationalism, etc. Utilitarianism, for example, deals with the idea of the greatest good for the greatest number. With absolutism, decisions are made from a fixed set of principles from which there is no deviation-the consequences of actions have no bearing on the decisions made. Rationalism relies upon previously set precedents and varies by circumstances. Situationalism involves an examination of circumstances in each situation.

However, these words seem to remain abstractions to the students. There are three distinct levels of moral reasoning and that each of these levels contains two stages:

a) Pre-conventional level:

— *Stage one*: The reward and punishment stage. We do what is right in order to avoid punishment.

— *Stage two*: The individualism and reciprocity stage. Although we still act out of self-interest, we recognise that other people have their interests also. Consequently, we enter into "deals" in order to secure our interests.

b) Conventional level:

— *Stage three*: The interpersonal conformity stage. We live up to what is expected of us by people close to us (family, friends) or by society in general.

— *Stage four:* The law and order or social system stage. We meet our obligations in order to keep the system as a whole going. Morality becomes a mere process of obeying the laws and rules of society.

c) Post-conventional level:

— *Stage five*: The social contract stage. We are concerned that laws and duties should be based on a rational calculation of overall utility (for example, the greatest good for the greatest number).

— *Stage six*: The universal principles stage. We believe in the validity of universal moral principles and have a sense of personal commitment to the values upon which those principles are based.

PROFESSIONAL AND ORGANISATIONAL ETHICS

Once students understand the ethical decision-making process, they are ready to approach the concept of a code of ethics-the idea that at times different groups of people establish very specific standards to govern very specific behavior. Codes of ethics are formalised social constructions that are agreed upon and/or imposed by social organisations (i.e. professional organisations, work organisations, and other such groups of people with a common purpose). It is helpful at this point to distinguish between a code of ethics and a code of behavior. A code of behavior can be written by any group wishing to distinguish its members from the rest of society. A code of behavior can refer to any type of behavior, whether or not the behavior impacts society.

A code of ethics, on the other hand, codifies the group's relationship to society. It must be consistent with the expectations of society; and, within those parameters, society must agree to allow the group the freedom to determine-specifically-what the group may do in its relationship to that society. Although Behrman articulates this idea, concerns with the relationship between society and the profession, and the profession's obligation to serve in the public interest, can be seen throughout the professionalism literature as well.

It is important for students to understand that a code of ethics is a critical part of an occupation's claim to professional status. Occupational groups develop codes of ethics for two primary reasons:

a) As a way to establish the standards of what will be expected of their members; and
b) To attain for their group the status of a profession, which is particularly important in emerging professions like public relations.

It is important to keep in mind that the status of a profession is particularly important to the professional's claim to autonomy-the right to retain the power to judge, define and practice the occupation in which he or she participates. Professionals justify their right to work autonomously, to be judged by their peers, to set the standards of their profession and many other privileges, by agreeing to work in the public interest-an agreement articulated in the profession's code of ethics.

In short, organisations frequently require employees including public relations professionals-to agree to follow their code of ethics-which often are codes of behavior. The organisational code of ethics frequently has to do with not disclosing corporate secrets that impact the organisation's profitability instead of or in addition to its relationship to society. This becomes an important element in the decision- making process and may at times conflict with the practitioner's professional code of ethics.

Again, the commitment to operate in the public interest is the essential criterion for a code of ethics.

By adhering to the PRSA Code of Professional Standards, public relations professionals agree to work in the public interest. What they do has an impact on society-people make important decisions based on what public relations practitioners do and say to influence powerful publics, such as the news media, stock market influentials, legislators, etc. Therefore, the obligation to work in the public interest is essential.

There are many professional organisations for public relations practitioners-the Public Relations Society of America and the International Association of Business Communicators, to name just a few. Each has a code of ethics; and, when viewed as a whole, what those codes have in common is the call for practitioners to be honest, to deal fairly with employers and employees, to inform accurately, to end relations with employers who request unethical conduct and to work in accord with the public interest. Codes of ethics incorporate pieces of the Kohlberg and Pagano models. However, whereas those models apply to the individual, codes of ethics, and even codes of behavior, set group norms that attempt to shape and are sometimes in conflict with individual norms.

Once students understand the concept of and reasons for ethical decision making, they need to face the complexity of making those decisions. Codes of ethics impose on the individual more than a simple system of professional "law and order"-they define for the individual how the stages of morality should be enacted in the professional arena. They do this not only for their own members or the members of their own profession, but for those who choose to interact with their members as well.

A primary example of this is the relationship between journalists and public relations practitioners. You might consider bringing in the Code of Ethics of the Society of Professional Journalists (SPJ) and have the students discuss the articles in the codes from SPJ and PRSA that either complement or conflict with each other. Understanding the publics of public relations (of which media are only one) also means understanding how these publics define their moral responsibility to society and are being responsive to their moral imperatives. This becomes particularly important in the global arena.

Students need to understand that codes of ethics are guideposts, not guarantees. Individuals make ethical decisions based on a variety of philosophical grounds, ranging from pragmatism to altruism. Making an ethical decision is a complex process of deliberation, rooted fundamentally in the individual, but lived out in a society that challenges him or her.

PRSA's Code of Professional Standards always looks so neat and pristine, yet its application is frequently so messy and complex. This is the students' opportunity to engage that complexity. Using case studies from the course textbook, the literature or your own experience, give the students a case developed around the PRSA code, or one of the other professional or organisational codes. Let them discuss in small groups how they would handle the situation you have presented. This works as well for groups of 15 as it does for groups of 150. When most of the groups appear to be winding down (15 minutes or so), call them back together and ask them to share their solutions.

Play devil's advocate-look for the holes in their arguments or present additional complications. If you are presenting a case history, give them the problem, let them solve it, then give them the solution the organisation in the case history developed and discuss the solution. Better yet, bring in credible practitioners who can present their own case studies. In advanced classes, where you have a number of students who have internship or other work experience behind them, let the students develop a case problem based on their encounters in the workplace. A good place to start is often right where they are-what are the ethics of being a student? Help them to see that they are building their ability to deal with increasingly complex ethical situations in their student lives.

11

BUILDING CORPORATE RESPONSIBILITY THROUGH PUBLIC RELATIONS

The International Youth Foundation (IYF) is one of the world's largest public foundations supporting programmes to improve the conditions and prospects for young people where they live, learn, work, and play. Path breaking in the mid – 1990s, strategic long-term collaborations among government, business, and civil society actors in the pursuit of common objectives are today a staple of the emerging global community. Yet while much has been said and written on the anticipated advantages of inter-sectoral partnering (ISP), it is only recently that a small but growing number of serious studies have begun to examine specific organisational experiences with this approach. Given its relative newness as an organisational strategy, even less has been written on the concrete results achieved at the project level, the relative value added of this approach versus others, or the systemic impact of ISP on relations among these three sectors.

Its mission is "to positively impact the greatest number of young people, in as many places as possible, in the shortest amount of time, with programmes that are effective, and in ways that are sustainable. " Designed to bring worldwide attention and resources to bear on a wide array of highly effective local efforts already transforming the lives of young people across the globe, IYF emphasises positive, holistic youth development strategies.

IYF focuses on the ways in which young people can improve their own conditions and those of the communities in which they live. Youth are viewed as protagonists rather than as passive recipients of assistance, and as doers rather than as victims of difficult circumstances. IYF and its global network of national, independent nonprofit youth organisations carry out activities in over 60 countries. Over the past decade, IYF and IYF Partners have helped more than 23 million young people gain access to the basic life skills, education, job training, and opportunities that are critical to their success.

ISP has been a key strategy of the Foundation from its inception and has become even more critical with the marked acceleration of IYF's partnering with the corporate sector over the last five years. With more global companies looking for ways to maximise their social investments, IYF is helping a growing number of the world's largest corporations implement customised social responsibility programmes in multiple countries. IYF looks carefully at both a company's giving interests and core business needs, matching those with international programmes of proven merit.

By executing branded programmes that improve prospects for young people all over the world, IYF helps corporations maximise their investments. Rather than build new programmes from scratch, IYF and IYF Partners target established programmes with strong track records and help to increase their reach. By linking national Partners to international investors and donors,

IYF helps to "scale up" best practice programmes – extending their benefits to greater numbers of young people. Recognising the pivotal role of its network in carrying out its mission, IYF invests considerable time and resources in expanding its local Partners' capacity and sustainability.

INTER – SECTORAL PARTNERING

ISP has emerged as a strategic approach to development, corporate responsibility, and citizen engagement at three levels: macro/global, sectoral, and organisational. It is useful to mention the distinct-though related-factors that fostered the rapid adoption of this approach at each level.

Macro/Global Level

IYF's adoption of a strategy of public-private partnering reflects similar developments taking place at the global level during the 1990s. Among the factors that created impetus for the exploration of new modes of institutional collaboration at the international level were the following:

- Increasingly complex, global development challenges (e. g., environment, health, economic growth) that transcended the capacity of any one sector-government, business or civil society-to resolve them.
- Growing resource constraints (particularly in terms of the ability of many governments to invest in critical social and economic development programmes) that underscored the need to mobilise new resources-human and financial.
- Strong corporate growth at the international level and related shifts in the way in which the business community and civil society viewed issues such as corporate social responsibility.

— Dramatic examples of democratic political opening that expanded the prospects for decentralisation and local empowerment, allowing local citizens to play a more active role in their own development.

— Burgeoning capacity and interest on the part of civil society actors around the world to take advantage of increased civic space in order to play a central role in development assistance.

— Emerging recognition of the need to build mutually reinforcing networks of inter-sectoral institutional arrangements at the local, national, and international levels to foster sustained development.

— Reduction in ideological differences with the end of the Cold War that in many places ushered in a new spirit of dialogue and cooperation among sectors historically at odds with one another.

— A revolution in information technology that fostered the flow of data across sectors and across regions and enhanced cross-sectoral thinking, organising, and collaboration.

— A global movement of information sharing and advocacy regarding corporate accountability that created social pressure and increased consumer awareness of corporate social responsibility issues.

As organisations began to collaborate, other more specific incentives to pursue ISP as an organisational strategy became apparent. ISP created opportunities for organisations to:

— Scale up initiatives.

— Increase their organisational capacity, visibility, and credibility.

— Take advantage of partner strengths as each sector brought a distinct set of core competencies to the table.

— Mobilise new resources.
— Lower costs and risks.
— Share information.
— Create new ideas/innovate.
— Leverage the political capital of ISP partners.
— Achieve a new range of outcomes.
— Share and build upon partner capacities, such as technical expertise.
— Better understand the different sectoral strengths and constraints of their partners.
— Build linkages across different communities.
— Provide a foundation for broader change.
— Foster indigenous philanthropy.
— Contribute to greater societal resilience.

Sectoral Level

In addition to these overarching trends, government, business, and civil society each have their own distinct sectoral motivations to pursue ISP arrangements.

Business

A healthy global economy, multinational corporations have demonstrated growing interest in expanding their corporate social responsibility (CSR) programmes in both developed and developing countries. No longer smallscale, ad hoc "good works" programmes, CSR initiatives are frequently signature programmes of major global corporations.

They are characterised by significant visibility within the global community and enjoy strong support among stakeholders (particularly employees) within the company. IYF's experience with ISP, IYF has formed a growing number of "outsourcing" partnerships with companies that are conducting their CSR work through civil society organisations.

Corporate motivations are varied, complex, and often met with skepticism on the part of some civil society actors. The need for corporate social responsibility (or as some refer to it, corporate citizenship) stems in large measure from the "New Economy" of speed, global reach, knowledge/intellectual capital, and branding.

Given that one quarter of the world's total wealth is tied up in 'brand value,appearing socially responsible is key, since brand value depends greatly on public perception. In addition to questions related to brand, corporations recognise the need to market their products and services to healthy, educated consumers with sufficient buying power. Similarly, they need access to a well-trained, healthy, and productive local work force.

CSR programmes that support development worldwide are directly related to longterm corporate success and sustainability. Specifically, ISP affords corporations multiple opportunities to:

— Outsource philanthropy to credible, reputable civil society organisations (CSOs) instead of investing their own human and financial capital in developing local networks of best practice programmes and securing top-notch technical expertise.

— Develop "cause branding," an increasingly important strategy for product/company differentiation in a saturated market, whereby businesses engage in longterm social commitments on specific causes that then become identified with the company's brand as a core component of organisational identity and corporate reputation.

— Attract employees by making the company a "preferred employer". Many studies show that job seekers will take a job with a socially responsible company over a similar position with a non-socially responsible company. Also, a socially responsible company has a degree of "insurance" or "glue" to keep morale high during hard times.

— Promote the company's specific industry and/or to fill a corporate need for human resources. These dual, value-added components can be seen clearly in the Cisco Systems Networking Academy programme, which both fills a need for trained technicians and serves to promote the IT sector as a whole.

  It is also at play as part of an American Express travel industry training programme that is a Global Partnership for Youth Development (GPYD) focus project in Brazil. Company sponsored school-to-work programmes have a high return on investment, as a recent analysis by the National Employer Leadership Council (NELC) confirms.

— Foster learning and innovation, finding new ways to solve problems and promoting a "learning company model". The "New Economy's" focus on knowledge, speed, innovation, and flexibility means that businesses able to incorporate the lessons learned from partnership experiences will be more successful than those that are not.

In sum, there has been an important and definitive shift from the "noblesse oblige" paternalistic corporate philanthropic model to the new corporate social responsibility (CSR) model, which posits the relationship between sectors not as a one-way financial transaction, but instead as a multi-level management strategy. Partnerships with CSOs and local government are part of this new paradigm.

Civil Society

Decreases in official development assistance, the privatisation of formerly public services, and linkages between corporate/business activities and human/community development concerns have contributed to growing CSO interest in ISP. There are a number of specific advantages for CSOs:

— *Funding and in-kind contributions*: Many CSOs are severely lacking in funds, making sustainability a significant problem. Inter-sectoral partnerships (ISPs)bring new, hitherto untapped resources to the development field.

— *Technical expertise*: This is particularly true in the case of youth employment, where the private sector is a key stakeholder. The market expertise and job placement opportunities that the business sector can provide are invaluable in assuring that YE programmes actually lead to jobs for young people. Neither the government nor civil society can create jobs by themselves, nor are these two sectors experts on market needs and fluctuations.

By the same token, the private sector needs government to promote an enabling environment for job creation and civil society expertise in youth development to prepare young people to be competent employees.

— Access to corporate networks and target groups such as young factory workers and local subsidiaries of multinationals. The ability to leverage relationships (which constitutes political and social capital) is expanded through partnership arrangements.

In terms of CSO/business partnering alone, corporations bring CSOs an infusion of intellectual capital, programmatic ideas, funding, networks, and leveraging power. Partnering with government may provide CSOs with the opportunity to take small-scale programmes to the regional or national level and/or to secure a critical change in national policy.

Government is a key player in promoting an "enabling environment" for ISPs. In many countries and regions of the world, government has convening power, credibility, and a command of resources that the corporate and/or CSO communities may lack. It therefore plays a particularly important role in creating an environment-policy, legal and regulatory mechanisms-conducive to development.

As many governments in both developed and developing countries faced growing resource constraints coupled with mounting development challenges (both nationally and at the international level) in the early to mid-1990s, they began to look for ways to devolve certain rights and responsibilities to the social sector and to the corporate sector. ISP began to attract growing attention.

The US Agency for International Development (USAID) was an early leader in this arena. Spurred by a declaration by Vice President Gore in March 1995 at the World Development Summit in Copenhagen, USAID launched the New Partnerships Initiative (NPI), an ambitious effort to develop a framework for strategic partnerships among government, business, and civil society actors that would link efforts to improve the international enabling environment for ISP with local empowerment.

The goal was to "provide local citizens with a legitimate role in the development process, a stake in its success, the capacity to act, and a clear sense of shared responsibility for the results." In the succeeding years, other organisations moved in this same direction. The Development Assistance Committee of the Organisation for Economic Cooperation and Development (OECD) developed a framework for cooperation among bilateral aid agencies; the World Bank launched the Comprehensive Development Framework (CDF); and the United Nations advanced the United Nations Development Assistance Framework (UNDAF).

This confluence of initiatives reflected an emerging consensus within the development assistance community that government, business, and civil society could work in partnership to take advantage of creative synergies and to achieve outcomes that would have been impossible for any one of them to achieve independently. Some of the incentives for ISP from the perspective of government include:

— Budgetary relief due to financial sponsorship by a corporate partner of services (e. g., job training) that otherwise would come from government funds.

— Access to the technical expertise, local contacts, and credibility of local CSOs.

— Economic, human development of community/ city/state/country.

— Enhanced enforcement of laws with the CSR model. For example, social clauses prohibiting child labour in supply chains help governments realise their commitments made as signatories of the Convention on the Rights of the Child (CRC).

Organisational Level

At the level of the individual organisation, motivations vary as well. IYF was an early pioneer in efforts to work collaboratively with both the public and private sectors, at times in tri-sectoral relationships. Senior management at IYF was quite intentional in its efforts to pursue such a strategy. IYF has consistently sought at all levels – in its international board and the boards of its affiliate national Partners – to promote the strong engagement of business leaders. It positioned itself from its founding to recruit global corporations to participate in and contribute to development projects. Furthermore, IYF has:

— Nurtured a relationship with the Financial Times (FT), which has lead to the biannual publication of a "Youth Survey".

— Engaged the World Economic Forum at its annual meeting in Davos, Switzerland.

— Consistently interacted with business groups and associations such as the International Chamber of Commerce (ICC) and the Conference Board.

It would seek to carry out such a mission through its intention to implement a global programme in over 60 countries, while simultaneously tailoring each national part of the programme to fit local needs and using local resources.

The "Irresistible Proposition" posits that IYF is an effective way for corporations and governments to invest in the world's youth, based on its extensive array of "best practice" partners and programmes, connections with some of the world's most influential leadership and "opinion-shapers" concerned with youth issues, and high international standards for financial responsibility, transparency, and accountability.

IYF's internal strategy for the promotion of ISP approaches is evidenced by its recruitment of a multilingual and multicultural staff with considerable experience working with private philanthropy, official development assistance programmes, non-profits, and the business world.

Other challenges with which some of the early ISP pioneers (particularly CSOs) struggled were: distrust, a fear of institutional "capture,"co-optation, and/or an inability to stick to mission due to power imbalances between sectors; self-doubt (many CSOs, for example, significantly underestimated the value of the experiences and expertise they would bring to an ISP); bureaucratic inertia in the face of changes in "standard operating procedures"; capacity deficits within a sector and/or an individual organisation; and differences in work style and expectations from one sector to the next.

Mainstreaming ISP

As organisations gained experience with ISP, the relationships among the partners and the nature of the partnerships themselves evolved and matured. Taken together with the results achieved, the challenges mentioned above were an impetus to revisit and refine roles and responsibilities and to begin to place greater emphasis upon questions of sustainability and the measurement of impact.

In the space of six years, for example, USAID's New Partnerships Initiative evolved. The ways in which USAID will work with nongovernmental organisations (including faith-based groups, private foundations, and universities) and the corporate sector at both the local and international level.

"Before, and in many cases still, you have a situation where one group-usually the non-profits-end up going 'door to door' with their proposal and asking the private sector or the government to buy it. " Non-profits are, however, not the only ones "selling. " In first generation ISP models, the government is using programmes to sell its policy agenda, the business sector to sell its marketing strategy, and civil society to sell its cause.

By the end of the 1990s, business (from multinationals to small and medium enterprises), government (at the international, national, and local levels), and the full array of civil society organisations (foundations, environmental groups, universities, religious organisations, etc.) began to view ISPs not as "special initiatives," but rather as staples of their organisational approaches.

Inter – sectoral Partnering

Youth development (YD) is an area that is particularly conducive to ISP arrangements. The adoption of the Convention on the Rights of the Child (CRC) by 191 countries in 1999has created a favorable climate for partnerships around this issue, providing governments with both a mechanism and a mandate to look for new ways to promote the rights of this often overlooked population.

Inter-sectoral partnerships in this arena are evolving even as the youth development field is still in the process of being defined, thus creating opportunities for innovation. It is only in the last two or three years that organisations such as the World Bank, USAID, and a number of private foundations, have begun to look at youth developmentas a discrete area of investment. Previously, youth were often dealt with in a more ad hoc, fragmented manner-as part of a health or education programme, for example.

Today, institutions are taking a more holistic approach to youth development. IYF has been able to take the lead in pairing an increasingly sophisticated partnership approach with an area of fast growing interest on the part of governments, corporations, and foundations. Not only are children and youth a non-threatening and emotionally satisfying area of corporate and/or foundation engagement, but the turn of the millennium added to global interest in "doing something for the next generation. "

From a corporate standpoint, it is difficult to think of a more attractive beneficiary population. Work on behalf of children and youth has a universal appeal that crosses political, religious, and ethnic lines. Focusing on youth and education is a natural fit for Nokia, a leader in future-oriented technologies.

In addition to its marketing benefits, the issue of improving the lives of children and youth is also a vital concern for corporate employees, who have their own families and can easily relate to the cause. Given earlier discussions on the advantages that corporate social responsibility programmes offer in terms of human resources, it is clear that strong employee buy-in and connection to corporate philanthropic ventures is highly desirable.

IYF AND ISP

IYF's emphasis on long-term youth development and its focus on the positive as opposed to the negative aspects of youth issues increases the organisation's attractiveness to potential ISP partners. At the same time, long-term outcomes of positive youth development are often harder to measure than the impact of child survival or disease prevention programmes.

Impact data that 1,000 children have been saved from polio via inoculation is much more easily gathered than data suggesting that 1,000 children have higher self-esteem due to holistic programming. The private sector wants to be able to document tangible, visible results, and while a focus on the positive is helpful from a marketing perspective, civil society must be able to demonstrate clear linkages between programming and these sometimes more intangible youth outcomes.

A second factor that increases IYF's attractiveness to corporate partners is the emphasis placed on local programmes rather than "cookie cutter" global programmes. Since the partnerships are designed and implemented by IYF's local Partner organisations, they are able to easily adapt to local cultures and communities.

Much in the same way as "glocal"companies have international brands and/or a series of products with substantial adaptation to local culture and surroundings,IYF has implemented global programmes based on general themes, but designed to match local circumstances. This facilitates the involvement of local corporate subsidiaries, allowing them to take ownership of the project and create ISPs on a local level.

Corporate employees volunteer for the programmes because it affects their community and their lives. This local emphasis significantly strengthens long-term sustainability and also reflects the idea that those closest to a problem are the best situated to find its solution. It is important to note that this experiment in ISP is a work in progress. IYF is on a steep and continual learning curve about how partnerships work and what the benefits and challenges are of such an approach.

The categories and conjectures presented here are not hard and fast, but are instead flexible, dynamic, and subject to change as new theories, evaluations, and practices emerge.

IYF's experience with ISP is primarily at the global level. While many isolated partnerships are initiated on a local case-by-case basis-for example, a local dry cleaner who buys uniforms for a community-based youth soccer league-IYF is one of the first civil society organisations to attempt the ISP approach transnationally.

Highlighted in this section are four global IYF partnerships: two represent tri-sectoral partnerships (business + civil society + government) and two represent bi-sectoral partnerships (business + civil society and government + civil society respectively). They offer the opportunity to examine partnering not only between local implementing institutions, but also at the highest levels, among companies, governments, and civil society organisations whose reach extends across the globe.

IYF has chosen to partner with a wide range of corporations-some that are relatively neutral in terms of their development reputation, such as Lucent Technologies and Nokia, and others who have been on the receiving end of significant public pressure like Nike, Shell, and Unocal. This reflects IYF's belief that all businesses have a role to play in promoting social responsibility.

For IYF, corporate social responsibility is best promoted by civil society having a "seat at the table" and the ability to engage the private sector as allies and partners in development. Additionally, IYF realises that it does not work in a vacuum-its partnerships with corporations are part of a continuum of strategies that seek to promote corporate responsibility. That continuum also includes other organisations that focus on advocacy, legislation, and accountability. The IYF initiatives highlighted in the following :

Global Alliance for Workers and Communities (GA)

The Global Alliance for Workers and Communities (GA) is a five-year, Rs. 12 crore programme that seeks to improve the workplace experience and life prospects of workers in the global manufacturing industry. The programme currently operates in China, India, Indonesia, Thailand, and Vietnam, where the vast majority of the workers are young women.

Through a rigorous, independent participatory assessment process by a local research institution (usually university affiliated), workers identify workplace issues and life aspirations. Personal development and training programmes are then developed that respond directly to workers' needs. The focus of the programme is on health services, personal financial services, vocational skills, educational opportunities, and life skills training. These services are delivered through local CSOs, including IYF's Partner organisation in Thailand.

Nike and Gap are both leaders in the corporate social responsibility field, in no small part because their success as businesses lies in the value of their brand. In the case of Nike, significant damage was done to its brand and sales after a series of media exposés on poor labour standards in its global supply chain. Instead of shying away from the issue, Nike has chosen to directly address the challenge by instituting compliance standards and publicising its efforts to improve labour practices throughout the supply chain.

The Body Shop, notes that one of the most powerful approaches a company can take in response to effective negative public campaigns is to partner with civil society organisations and thereby directly address the issue at hand. Due to its youth development focus and the expertise of the various partners, the GA offers companies an opportunity to go beyond monitoring activities and engage in sustainable development initiatives based on partnership.

Additionally, civil society involvement lends credibility to a company's corporate responsibility strategies. For IYF, the Global Alliance provides access to a significant segment of the population of young people-young factory workers-who might otherwise not have access to traditional youth development programmes and services.

The government component – represented in this partnership by the World Bank – provides substantial research and policy input, including critically important country situational analysis and ongoing policy dialogue between country representatives and local government. Additionally,World Bank involvement has led to a potential pilot in which the International Finance Corporation (IFC) may develop a personal finance programme for workers.

Global Partnership for Youth Development (GPYD)

The Global Partnership for Youth Development (GPYD) is part of the World Bank's Business Partners for Development (BPD) programme that seeks to identify and learn from new forms of partnership that relate business interests and social and human development needs.

GPYD was launched in 1999 and has a three-fold mission: to identify and disseminate what works in tri-sectoral partnering for youth development; to mobilise new resources; and to invest in scaling up and strengthening best practice. Several of the focus projects are implemented in collaboration with IYF national Partner organisations and have resulted in project case studies in Thailand, the Philippines, Poland, and Brazil.

Most of the GPYD programmes focus on youth employment and/or education initiatives, which lend themselves particularly well to an ISP approach. Governments, for example, are concerned with unemployment rates because they can add to economic and social instability and may be particularly costly in nations where there is state-funded welfare.

Businesses are interested in access to the best-trained workforce possible with skills appropriate and desirable to the market. CSOs are aware of the vital importance of employment for young people-not only because it alleviates poverty and combats social exclusion, but also because of the life skills and selfesteem gained through the opportunity to contribute productively to one's community.

Yet government and CSOs alone cannot create jobs, and the private sector has neither the experience nor the expertise to deal with the comprehensive developmental issues that come into play when providing job training for disadvantaged youth. The private sector can, however, provide information as to what kinds of skills are needed in the market and an "in" to the world of work via internships and job placement.

Government and CSOs can take the lead in providing training programmes, teaching young people not only the technical skills they need, but also the life skills that are vital to the workplace of the 21st century.

Nokia

The Nokia Make a Connection programme is a multi-year global programme to support initiatives aimed at helping youth "make a connection" with their communities, families and peers, and themselves through youth participation and life skills training. The programme is currently operating in eight countries (Brazil, China, Germany, Mexico, Poland, the Philippines, South Africa, and the United Kingdom) and is expected to expand to several more in the coming years.

The global component includes YouthActionNet. org, a website providing information, inspiration, and tools for young people actively engaged in contributing to their communities and a series of What Works publications produced by the IYF Learning and Evaluation Department. Make a Connection is the signature component of Nokia's corporate social responsibility programme and a key partnership for IYF in its efforts to build alliances with the corporate sector for the benefit of child and youth development.

The Nokia – IYF partnership is an excellent example of how outsourcing to a network of youth-serving organisations with proven expertise and reach is a highly effective way for corporations to invest in young people. As a leader in the corporate social responsibility field, Nokia was convinced of the "natural fit" between its future-oriented strategy and investing in child and youth development.

Rather than create its own foundation and/or spend its philanthropic dollars developing the expertise or the bureaucracy to handle philanthropic initiatives, Nokia chose to partner with IYF. In this way, Nokia was able to invest in youth with low infrastructure and overhead costs and IYF was able to bring new resources to the field as well as facilitate relationships with Nokia subsidiaries at a local level, thereby laying the groundwork for a strengthened grassroots public/private sector collaboration on child and youth development.

As one Nokia executive said, it was an opportunity to combine "valuebased leadership" with "factbased management. "Eventually, the goal of both IYF and Nokia is to have the local subsidiaries take full ownership of the programme, financially and otherwise. In this way, development strategies are implemented by partnerships between local business and community organisations that have a stake and presence in the community and are therefore more invested in its social and economic welfare.

The local subsidiary involvement also shows the multiplier effect of ISP using global networks to create local partnerships. Through this larger international collaboration, the local CSOs in the IYF Partner Network have access to key in-country corporate contacts.

Nokia and IYF staff communicate regularly about programme status and updates, discuss trends and challenges, and work together to resolve problems quickly and effectively. Throughout the process, difficult issues are addressed directly. One such issue was the intermittent tension that would appear when local Nokia staff and local IYF Partners would find they had different professional judgments about how to improve the prospects of young people.

Other issues included Nokia's desire to allow its employees greater opportunities to play a direct, voluntary role in these programmes. In a departure from traditional checkbook philanthropy, Nokia staff are enthusiastic about contributing directly to service delivery at the local level. Through numerous conversations among the partners, these differences in perspective were resolved.

Entra 21

The IYF-MIF collaboration is a four year Rs. 24 crore programme to improve the employability of 12,000 disadvantaged youth, ages 14 to 29 in Latin America and the Caribbean. A fundamental aspect of the programme is mobilising private sector investment in terms of funding, job training, and job placement.

Approximately 35-40 grants will be given to model projects to promote private sector partnerships, gender equity, sustainability, and capacity strengthening of implementing organisations. Training for information technology (IT) in the workplace and job placement services are included, as well as a significant learning and dissemination component.

Economic stability in Latin America and the Caribbean is a major focus of the Inter-American Development Bank. In a region where unemployment rates are frequently over 30% and where youth account for approximately 50% of the population, there is a pressing need to tackle economic issues from a child and youth development angle.

In light of the IT revolution, it is clear that countries boasting a workforce trained in knowledge, communications, and information skills will attract the coveted IT business that has become a benchmark of global competitiveness. However, the key question is how to use the potential of IT to help close the existing divides between rich and poor within national boundaries.

IYF, for its part, is very concerned with the growing digital divide and how it can lead disadvantaged youth, already suffering from societal exclusion, further and further behind. Entra 21 combines the youth development expertise and grassroots service delivery network of IYF with the economic market expertise, convening power, and financial resources of the IDB.

To facilitate the involvement of the private sector, the MIF grant is a one-to-one challenge requiring that an additional $10 million be raised through business partnerships, particularly with IT companies. The programme will therefore quickly become a tri- as opposed to bi-sectoral partnership.

IYF Partners and ISP

The programmes described above involve global actors from civil society, business, and government. Equally important to study are initiatives that are locally based. For this reason, this section details the experiences of six IYF Partners engaged in "on the ground" work with the inter-sectoral partnership model.

Some of the local ISPs described here are part of the larger, global relationships listed above. Some are locally initiated. All are tri-sectoral and represent different aspects of how, why, where, and to what effect ISP is being used in the field.

Model for ISP Advocacy

The Child Friendly Company (CFC) programme was initiated by Fundação Abrinq as part of its mission to eradicate child labour in Brazil. It uses traditional advocacy and lobbying coupled with ISP to advance the cause of child rights. The programme provides a "Child Friendly Company (CFC)" seal, which corporations may apply for and, if accepted, use on their products.

The guidelines for what constitutes a CFC include no child labour at any level in the production/supply chain and a philanthropic commitment to child and youth development. Applications undergo a due diligence process and the corporations must reapply annually. In addition to the seal, the programme works on promoting social clauses in business contracts, particularly in the charcoal (and therefore motor vehicle), sugar-alcohol, footwear, and citrus fruit production and supply chains.

Fundação Abrinq is particularly interested in influencing federal, state, and municipal policies around child labour issues and the reintegration of children and youth in the formal school system. It was key in lobbying for the passage of the Convention on the Rights of the Child in Brazil and plays a major role in the inter-sectoral National Forum for Eradication of Child Labour (FNETI).

The eradication of child labour requires a significant degree of collaboration with the private sector. The question is how willingly the private sector cooperates. Critics charge that ISPs allow corporations to project a good image through their association with respected civil society actors, thereby legitimising their business while changing little in corporate policy or substantially improving their environmental or social practices.

This marketing diversion tactic has been termed "green washing" by the global environmental movement. Recent corporate partnerships with UN agencies have led to a new term, based on the colour of the UN flag- "blue washing." The Abrinq model shows that while "green and bluewashing" does occur, ISPs can also be used to reward those companies that act responsibly while "forcing the hand" of those that do not.

Abrinq practices traditional advocacy with a twist, excelling at the rather difficult task of combining both public awareness and confrontational strategies with the newer partnership approach. Companies that apply for the seal tend to do so for three reasons: to gain recognition for the philanthropic activities they are already involved in with children and youth; for social marketing purposes or to improve their image; and as future "insurance" for demanding customers that helps to differentiate them from other companies making similar products.

For example, a sugar cane company, which suffers from that industry's historical association with slavery and plantation- style production, puts the seal on its invoices and sugar sacks. Paratodos, a bus company involved in the programme, displays the seal on all its buses. The highprofile visibility of the seal produces a ripple effect in the business sector; once one company in the industry has it, others begin to apply for it in order to remain competitive.

In addition, since the seal requires a philanthropic commitment to children and youth, it promotes additional local level public/private partnerships. Paratodos, for example, runs a mobile museum for school children as part of a partnership between the company, public schools, and the São Paulo Modern Art Museum (MAM).

In terms of social clauses and policy, while some industry groups quickly joined the anti-child labour campaign, such as the Brazilian Association of Citrus Fruit Exporters (ABECITRUS), others required a sustained advocacy effort on the part of the civil society sector. It was signed by the Sugar-Alcohol Chamber of São Paulo, the Association of Sugar and Alcohol Industries in the State of São Paulo (AIAA), and the Abrinq Foundation, among others.

Through both the seal and the social clause projects, Abrinq has created the Network of Child Friendly Corporations REAC), which boasts over 2,000 members. The benefits of Abrinq's work with the government and private sector have been manifold. A National Protocol for the Eradication of Child Labour in Brazil was signed by Brazilian president Fernando Henrique Cardoso, ministers of State, 12 governors, members of Congress, business organisations, workers associations, and the Abrinq Foundation-underscoring how Abrinq has moved the issue to the forefront of federal policy.

Paisajoven

PaisaJoven (PJ) originated from a proposal made by the Medellín municipal government to the Deutsche Gesellschaft fur Technische Zusammenarbeit (German Agency for Technical Cooperation - GTZ) to fund a programme to combat high levels of youth unemployment in the city. Medellín, a Colombian city in the department of Antioquia, has been one of the "hot spots" of the drug violence and civil war that has plagued the country for over 50 years.

This insecurity has led to high levels of unemployment, high dropout rates, and an environment of antagonism and distrust among the government, business, and civil society sectors. In the PaisaJoven project, however, all three sectors were invited to design and participate in the project from its inception.

A tri-sectoral coalition oversaw the process by which it evolved into an independent non-profit organisation dedicated to facilitating the effectiveness of youth programmes by providing technical assistance and organisational capacity building, and promoting collaboration among different youth development actors through the creation of a network. The decision to create an organisation dedicated to institutional strengthening as a response to youth unemployment was both innovative and controversial.

During the planning stages, the groups split into two factions; one wishing to create a CSO dedicated exclusively to employment generation and the other to the formation of a network for institutional support for organisations already working with youth. The latter idea prevailed based on a pre-planning diagnosis of the situation by local experts that pointed to the main problems in the CSO working context.

It found that there was too much action without planning, a "reign of informality"/lack of professionalisation of the field, the tendency to view work with young people paternalistically in terms of "salvation and sacrifice," and a distinct lack of coordination among groups. PJ focuses on three main areas: employment, community development, and education. There are currently 50 members of the network, representing the business, government, and civil society sectors.

Paisa Joven is an interesting example of tri-sectoral partnering because all of the partners are local Colombian institutions. The business members are indigenous

Colombian companies, not larger multinational corporations. It is also noteworthy that during PaisaJoven's creation, one of the principal criteria for its institutional design was the participation of all three social sectors.

The argument for business involvement hinged on the view that the state could not directly create employment alone. At the same time, the governmental role would be vital in creating a favorable climate for local employment creation. Recognition of the need to include business, civil society, and government from the beginning was a result of GTZ's 25 years of experience, which had taught them that an initiative is only sustainable if it is created in the same country where it will be implemented and if it responds to needs identified by all local stakeholders living the reality of the situation.

Former executive director of Paisa Joven and one of the founding staff members, notes that involving all sectors was key given the specific goals and objectives of the organisation, namely to build social capital and encourage collaboration. In Medellín, where violence and political upheaval are the norm rather than the exception, it was clear that the original idea of housing the initiative in the mayor's office would subject it to the vagaries of Colombian politics.

Creating an organisation that was city and sector wide was, above all, a strategy for impact and sustainability. Young Minds in Motion-Poland,started in 1999, is a two-year project with the goal to equip schools in rural northeast Poland with computer hardware and software, while providing teacher training to raise the educational standards of the region. The regions in which the programme has been implemented, Barciany and Korsze, are two of the poorest in the country, suffering from high rates of unemployment, low educational levels, rural isolation, and various social problems including alcoholism.

Poland has undergone a dramatic transformation over the past twenty years. The opportunity for citizen participation and collaboration with the private sector has opened up as well as the need for civil society to "fill in the gaps" for public social services like education, employment, and healthcare that previously fell under the governmental social safety net.

Rural and impoverished people are the hardest hit by the loss of the federal safety net and employment and, while civil society is rapidly taking responsibility for meeting many social needs, the sector is still young and relatively under-funded. Additionally, the private sector is also in its infancy and has not fully articulated a "corporate social responsibility" ethic at this stage in its development.

To address these evolving changes in economic, social, and political systems, an ISP approach was adopted. PCYF provided funds via the World Bank and a Microsoft grant for hardware and teacher training, while the local municipalities agreed to subsidise electricity, additional telephone lines, and other infrastructure costs.

The local Microsoft Polish subsidiary office distributed software and provided the necessary licensing agreements to all participating schools. The programme has allowed municipal officials, parents, and teachers to combine resources and collaboratively create new approaches to development.

The computer labs placed in schools are also available for community use and have resulted in information technology (IT) training courses for unemployed adults, sponsored by the Ministry of Unemployment. Additionally, several youth groups successfully applied for and received grants from Polish CSOs to carry out youth – led projects in community and school service projects after participating in a leadership training workshop that was part of the pilot stage of the programme planning.

The resources provided by Microsoft were made useful as a result of the partnership among schools, municipal authorities, and the community. Perhaps most importantly, the project has created a collaborative and participatory self-help mindset, which has led to manifold spin-off projects and unexpected outcomes.

Cisco Systems

Cisco Systems created the Cisco Network Academy Programme (Networking Academy) in 1998 to provide training on computer network design, construction, and maintenance. As of 2001, the programme operates in 5,000 institutions in 84 countries, training over 129,000 people.

As in other parts of the world, the Philippine Cisco Networking Academies are the result of a tri-sectoral partnership among several national institutions. A focus project for GPYD, the Philippine programme seeks to enhance opportunities for out-of-school disadvantaged youth, who represented an estimated 16-39 percent of the youth population in 1998.

Young people trained in the academies, which function usually via already established educational institutions (in this case CITE and LaCAT), are eligible for certification as Cisco Certified Networking Associates. The key to the international growth of the Cisco Networking Academies programme has been its ability to partner with local institutions.

The original idea was developed out of a need to increase the pool of properly trained technicians due to the global shortage of IT workers, which was recently estimated by the International Data Corporation at one million. Coupled with this is the growth of the "New Economy" wherein companies have complex relationships not only with shareholders, but also with stakeholders-including local communities.

Cisco's desire to make "global to local" connections and to work with traditionally disadvantaged populations has made it an attractive partner for CSOs and governments trying to figure out how to more equitably distribute the skills, wealth, and opportunities presented by the emergence of the IT industry.

For the Children and Youth Foundation of the Philippines (CYFP) and the government's Department of Social Welfare and Development, the programme represents one way to attempt to bridge the digital divide between haves and have-nots and to combat youth unemployment and social exclusion by matching education/training to labour market demands.

However, the Philippine academies programme has gone a step beyond simply providing youth with marketable skills in recognition of the fact that the "skills gap" for IT workers not only refers to technical ability, but also to "softer skills" like creativity, communication, and teamwork. As a result of the CSO partners' expertise in youth development, a strong life skills curriculum-Skills for Life: A Programme Guide-was developed to strengthen communication, decision-making, problem solving, and goal-setting skills.

Rural Youth Career Development Programme

The Rural Youth Career Development Programme was originally initiated by the National Council on Youth Development (NCYD) as a response to the migration of youth from urban centers back to rural areas after Thailand's national economic crisis in 1997. It seeks to create career opportunities for young people by offering alternatives in the agricultural field and to encourage entrepreneurship and the revival of the rural agricultural community.

Focused in the northeastern area of the country, the programme provides a cohesive training package that includes vocational, management, marketing, and entrepreneurial skills, as well as small seed loans to graduates. One innovative aspect of the programme is that the young people are given an array of information on different potential agricultural careers and are then able to specialise in those of greatest interest to them.

The partnership between NCYD and Shell Thailand is a result of the international partnership between IYF and Shell International, which is in turn part of the Global Partnership for Youth Development (GPYD). It is a good example of "glocal" relationship as previously defined. Shell International provided funding for the programme through Shell-Thailand, although the national subsidiary did not actually provide any direct financial support.

However, Shell Thailand did use its connections in the business and government sectors to bring other companies and agencies into the project, including the Thai Cement Company and the Community Development Department of the Ministry of the Interior. Federal governmental agencies were key in ensuring the sustainability of the project and have replicated it through a Non-Formal Education Department joint project with the Bank for Agriculture.

Though national level partnerships played an active management role in this initiative, it is critical also to highlight the effect of tri-sectoral collaboration at the local level. In the target area of Sri Saket, for example, a community youth leader has successfully integrated the project into the sub-district local government (TAO) budget, thereby connecting the commitment of the national government to local government budgets. As in the Polish example, this points to the various unintended outcomes and increases in local ISP that often result from global or national partnership programmes.

Speak Out

Speak Out! (SO) was the brain child of The Body Shop-Australia (TBS-A), a national franchise holder of The Body Shop-International (TBS-I), whose mission is "to dedicate our business to the pursuit of social and environmental change. " SO is an independent T-shirt and "street wear" manufacturer that provides transitional employment and training for disadvantaged youth.

The idea for the programme was generated by TBS-A's dual objectives of finding uniforms for employees that were made under ethical labour conditions and working with youth, who make up a sizable portion of their clients and employees. SO is a non-profit organisation and is working towards self-sustainability through the sale of its products.

From the outset, TBS-A specifically sought out community and government involvement in the initiative and garnered the support of the Foundation for Young Australians (FYA) and the federal Department of Employment, Training, and Youth Affairs (DEETYA).

While TBS-A provides the physical infrastructure and leads the programme's overall development, the partnership has strengthened several aspects of SO. Some results of the partnership have been that young people are more effectively recruited through FYA youth programmes and DEETYA employment agencies; the programme is better equipped to handle life skills and other issues outside the purview of traditional business skills training; and the programme has been used as a model for best practice and replication throughout FYA's national and international network.

It is also important to note that TBS-A's social enterprise business model is a direct result of the corporate culture and strategies promoted by TBS-I. This is an excellent example of the effect international companies can have on their local subsidiaries.

Culture, Communication, and Compatibility

The public and private sectors have distinctly different "cultures" arising primarily from the fact that each sector has developed structures, vocabulary, and behaviours to best meet its own particular goals and objectives. While specific project goals may be compatible, the overall goal of a for-profit venture is necessarily different from that of a non-profit.

Carol Bellamy, Executive Director of UNICEF, in an address focusing on the UN's decision to promote private/public partnerships, stated that, "It is dangerous to assume that the goals of the private sector are somehow synonymous with those of the United Nations, because they most emphatically are not. "For this reason, a certain amount of "cultural translating" must take place in order to facilitate collaboration among groups.

There is a good deal of time that must be spent ensuring that all partners are on the same page. This is important not only in terms of issues such as the speed of business and management styles, but also in terms of ideological goals.

Flexibility: True strategic partnerships (as compared to traditional donor-grantee relationships) are not fixed entities, but function in a more fluid, cyclical manner. Different partners will take on different roles at various points in the programme cycle. The partnership itself may be shorter or longer than initially anticipated. In some cases it is formed simply to address an immediate, specific problem.

In other cases, it may lead to a long-term partnership or a permanent new organisation like PaisaJoven. Occasionally, not all the partners who began a project end up able or willing to remain partners throughout the programme. This was the case in the Thai example, where one of the business partners had to discontinue its involvement in the project. A partnership must be flexible and adaptable enough to deal with these unpredictable events, since business and civil society actors are subject to distinct external influences while government is subject to the vagaries of political life.

Flexibility applies not only to the ability to respond to external influences, but also to internal management and to the mindset of each partner. The Thai example proves instructive in this regard. Partners were willing to have meetings late in the evening if schedules did not allow for meetings during the day and to make field trips to project sites on the weekend.

In terms of attitude, then, there was a respect for differing organisational cultures and a willingness to compromise that is essential for successful ISPs. The Rural Youth Career Development programme published by the GPYD found that while Shell Thailand was punctual and focused on clear planning leading to measurable numerical results, the company cut down on some criteria and regulations in order to allow for NCYD's (the civil society partner) need for time and space to experiment with implementation strategies so as to find best practices.

The key government partner, the Department of Non Formal Education (NFE), "would have preferred to take the lead role of this project and to have the project as its showcase," but eschewed ownership in the interest of a more collaborative learning process.

Speed: Corporations tend to move quickly and to be more concerned with immediate results than the civil society sector, which tends to give considerable time to issues of process and long-term outcomes. This is evidenced in the case of the Cisco global academies programme. Business speed is generally faster than CSO speed, but e-business speed is off the charts. When one is dealing with IT training programmes, for example, the programme must work at the speed of technological development.

Cisco Systems, the business partner and founder of the Cisco Networking Academies programme, has found this issue of pace compatibility intermittently frustrating. For example, semi-annual university programme review meetings can interfere with the need to keep training, hardware, software, and facilities current in an industry where, according to Moore's law, the power of microprocessors doubles every 18 months.

Power Balance: One of the major challenges in public/ private partnering is the propensity, consciously or unconsciously, for the business partner to become the dominant force in decision-making. This is due to various factors including business management style and the fact that the financial resources that business brings may cause both public and private sector partners to fall into the more traditional "donor-recipient" mode wherein the donor is the entity providing the terms of cooperation.

However, as Darcy Ashman of the Institute for Development Research (IDR)points out, "corporate citizenship is not likely to produce significant development results unless CSOs are empowered partners". For this reason, there needs to be clear and equal value given to the resources that CSO and government partners bring to collaborative ventures, as well as a respect for the different management cultures of all three sectors.

Another way in which power imbalance is avoided is through partnerships like the Abrinq and PaisaJoven examples, where the resources provided by the business partner do not include money. These partnerships are based more on the human and social capital that the private sector brings in the form of employee volunteers, technical expertise, relationships with other businesses and/or governmental actors, the capacity for high profile publicity and marketing, etc.

Trust and Transparency: There must be active engagement of all partners in a transparent process. The best partnerships are those where there is an easy give and take among the parties. All partners can then participate fully from the design stage through evaluation and the distillation of lessons learned. Participation, communication and transparency are the essential building blocks of trust, and trust and mutual respect are the sine qua non of effective inter-sectoral partnerships.

Nike could have felt unfairly attacked and IYF could have withdrawn its decision to partner with the corporation. Instead, the relationship between the organisations led to considerable internal discussion and commitment to action, wide public dissemination of the report,the equally public commitment of Nike to a remediation plan to confront the issues raised, and a further cementing of the partnership relationship.

Issue Areas: Some development issues lend themselves especially well to ISP because the goals of all three sectors are particularly compatible.Youth development occupies a privileged niche in terms of its attractiveness to all three sectors. This "fit" is further strengthened when the specific youth development programme is unusually well-suited to a multi-sector approach, as in the case of employment, education, and the "digital divide."

Youth Employment: Few issues in the youth development arena are as clearly suited to an ISP approach as youth employment. It combines the interest of the government in a stable economy with the need of the business sector for a qualified workforce and the goals of youth-serving organisations of social inclusion and meaningful contribution for young people.

Speak Out, the Australian programme, and the Philippine Cisco System Networking Academy, are excellent examples. In fact, relative to other issue areas, there is an abundance of tri-sectoral projects dealing with youth unemployment and employability precisely because the connections among the sectors on this issue are so readily apparent. While youth employment per se may not be a "core business goal," businesses benefit substantially from positive youth employment outcomes and are able to contribute to these outcomes vis-à-vis their role as employers.

Education: Education is also a natural fit with an ISP approach, particularly public education. Not only does it require the involvement of government, but it is also a good way to involve corporate employees as volunteers, as many of them are parents and have children in the formal school system. The examples of ISP in schools listed above includes the Microsoft Young Minds in Motion programme, where the impact of education-based partnerships on local communities is most clearly demonstrated.

However, while education is in many ways an attractive area for ISP, it is also important to safeguard against situations in which some businesses can use schools and school children in unethical ways.

Digital Divide: The booming "New Economy" based on the information and communications technology (ICT) revolution has contributed to a digital divide between both rich and poor countries and among social classes within countries. It has also created hitherto unparalleled potential for all sectors to exchange information and ideas.

For young people, naturally inclined towards technology, the ICT boom could provide the skills necessary to succeed in a globalised world-if they have the opportunity to learn them. With a worldwide deficit in trained ICT workers of more than one million, according to the International Data Corporation, businesses and education systems alike are eager to encourage the acquisition of technical skills by children and youth.

Civil society sees an opportunity to open doors for traditionally disadvantaged populations and to help stem the increasing gaps in technological access. This is the impetus for the entra 21 programme promoting technological skills for youth in Latin America.

Advocacy: Other issue areas may require CSO advocacy in order to motivate partnerships with the private sector. Abrinq's Child Friendly Company programme is a prime example of how even issues that may be controversial can still be fertile ground for ISP. This is in line with the idea expressed by Jane Covey from the Institute of Development Research (IDR), who noted at the USAID Development Dialogue in April 2000 that, "Nonprofits should be willing to pressure business into joining in partnership with them, and they should be able to use advocacy if business is not willing to join. "

Regional and Country Settings: Organisations active in global inter-sectoral partnering must take into account both regional context and a country's specific economic, political, and social situation. What a partnership looks like in Poland is likely to be quite different from how it may look in Brazil or South Africa or India.

In Poland's fledgling private sector, there is not yet the emphasis on corporate social responsibility that there is in Brazil. In El Salvador, a long history of corrupt government has left a legacy of distrust wherein ISPs are unlikely to include government for a long time to come. In countries like India and the Philippines, with a long history of philanthropy, business people may often take the lead in ISP, although it may be seen more as financial "noblesse oblige" with less emphasis (at least initially) on the potential benefits it may bring to their enterprises.

Regional and national differences in terms of ISP are complex, depending on factors ranging from the relative sophistication of the private sector to the policy environment towards civil society to the specific social problems faced. In any region, a thorough examination must be made of each sector to determine if ISP is an appropriate and/or effective way of promoting development and solving problems.

History: The history of relations among the three sectors is critical to whether an ISP would or would not be able to achieve meaningful results. For example in some regions, such as Central America, civil war in the 1980s led to deep-seated distrust towards the government, meaning that government and civil society partnerships were unlikely to receive public support. In other regions, such as the former Soviet republics, civil society and the business sector are relatively new and the relationships are still evolving.

IYF has found that corporations tend to focus philanthropic programmes in their major market areas, which means that there is a need for global CSOs to think creatively about how to channel resources to countries and regions that may not be the private sector's top priority.

Due to the tendency for corporations and foundations alike to limit their investments to select countries, IYF is particularly interested in addressing the needs of IYF Partners that are not beneficiaries of major foreign investment from the private sector, and therefore is exploring the creation of a Global Development Fund within IYF.

This could be funded in part by allocating a small percentage of revenues that have been leveraged through IYF's corporate outsourcing efforts to countries that would not otherwise benefit from IYF's outsourcing role. IYF recognises the challenges of raising revenue for this purpose, but believes the Fund has the potential to attract support from a variety of donors-both corporate and nonprofit-that share concerns about the growing social and economic inequities worldwide.

IYF's partnerships with bilateral development assistance agencies and foundations that support activities in all parts of the world are another promising approach to the diversification of resources across the globe.

Global and Local Corporate Culture: Another issue when dealing with global programmes is the difference between international companies, which tend to have highly developed corporate social responsibility strategies, and national subsidiaries, which vary country to country in terms of their understanding of and commitment to solving development problems.

It is here that cultural values play a major role, whether they manifest themselves as a traditional "noblesse oblige" or "sacrifice" paradigm stemming from religious beliefs (as in Latin America)or a lack of an ethic of private sector service due to the relative newness of the market (as in Eastern Europe). This, however, also works both ways. Speak Out! is an excellent example of how the company culture of the international corporation can also affect the corporate social responsibility strategies of the local subsidiary.

Scale: As seen in the profile of the Nokia/IYF Make a Connection programme, one benefit to global programmes is the multiplier effect that international companies and global civil society organisations can have on partnerships between local CSOs and corporate subsidiaries. In turn, these local subsidiaries and CSOs often have their own networks of indigenous businesses and community groups to bring to the table.

Scaling up is facilitated when partners can tap into: civil society's extensive networks at both the international and (particularly) the grassroots level; global corporate linkages and their relationships with local subsidiaries; and the extensive resources and reach of national governments.

Policy: A country's enabling environment (in terms of the policy, legal, and regulatory frameworks) plays a critical role in the formation and sustainability of partnerships. The question of whether or not a country has adopted the Convention on the Rights of the Child and whether, for example, there is legislation (in the form of tax breaks, incentives, and mandatory social clauses, etc.) that allows the civil society sector to flourish and corporations to engage in philanthropy are key.

Noting that the shift from authoritarian to democratic regimes in Brazil and South Africa allowed previously censored CSOs to criticize corporate practices openly, Darcy Ashman finds that "as a consequence, the Brazilian and South African companies and their foundations were under pressure to demonstrate social responsibility and, in the South African case, comply with the law."

Transaction Costs: Transaction costs-which refers to the time and energy it takes to ensure that ISP members are talking the same language, building the capacity of each sector to understand and work effectively with other sectors, and the creation of personal relationships can be very high. There may be times where the costs outweigh the relative benefits of the approach.

This is particularly true when the problem to be addressed could be solved/handled by one sector as (or even more) effectively. It is also an issue when one sector is particularly weak and would require significant capacity building to reach the point where it could function as an equal partner with another, more developed sector. In such a situation, issues of time and cost must be weighed against the longterm value of strengthening that sector.

Compatibility of Goals: Partnerships work best when goals are compatible. Some civil society and government institutions specifically charged with serving the public good (such as the UN and the World Health Organisation) need to maintain a certain distance from private interests to do their job effectively. A recent World Health Organisation (WHO) report notes how tobacco companies have influenced the WHO by developing and maintaining relationships with key staff members and even putting tobacco industry consultants in positions at the WHO.

There is also the longstanding criticism made of the Codex Alimentarius Commission, a tri-sectoral partnership set up by the WHO in 1963 to establish food safety and quality standards but which includes several private sector representatives of the food industry as part of its decision-making body. There are clearly potential goal compatibility and conflict of interest issues involved in these examples of relationships between private industry and civil society organisations.

Social Pressure: Inter-sectoral partnerships constitute one part of a broad array of strategies to promote corporate social responsibility. Voluntary initiatives that businesses undertake as part of their CSR programmes are to be applauded as a complement to, not a substitute for, legislation and traditional advocacy. As the Abrinq example clearly shows, there is no need to "throw the baby out with the bathwater"-the voluntary participation in the CFC programme is an adjunct to the policy advocacy the foundation engages in on a national level.

Several ISP observers and practitioners postulate that pressure by civil society advocacy groups, such as during the Seattle protests of the World Trade Organisation (WTO) or the United Students Against Sweatshops (USAS) campaign against Nike, created a favorable climate for inter-sectoral partnerships between public and private entities. The social pressure facilitates the initial and sustained involvement of business in partnerships with civil society and government.

INTERMEDIARY ORGANISATIONS

IYF performs a significant intermediary role, linking civil society organisations, businesses, and governments. In the process, IYF identifies "what works," brings it to scale, and makes the case for youth to the broadest possible audience. It mobilises new resources at the global level-particularly within the corporate community and makes them available to some of the best youth development programmes around the world.

Similarly, IYF works with its local partners to expand their reach and build their capacity through the creation of a global network of youth development partners, resource mobilisation, technical support, and shared analysis of best practice. To date, IYF has concentrated on playing an outsourcing role with companies-particularly large multinationals-but is expanding that role to include a growing number of governments, foundations, and nonprofits who wish to support global children's programmes.

IYF's experience with the Global Alliance for Workers and Communities underscores the importance of a sense of collective responsibility and commitment to the stated (and evolving) objectives of a partnership. In early ISP initiatives, it was typical for each sector to feel most committed to and responsible for ensuring that its own objectives be met no matter what else happened. As relationships evolved and trust levels grew, however, there was an emerging recognition that the goals of ISPs are much more than the sum of the parts.

Over time, each sector begins to develop a commitment to a broader set of goals that reflect the interests of all members of the partnership as well as a collective (and perhaps public) interest. As IYF's President, Rick Little, has stated, "We expect to increase significantly our various partnerships with global companies and become one of the principal "outsourcing" vehicles through which multinational companies implement their agendas for corporate social responsibility.

IYF's focus would be on serving our mutual interests by developing comprehensive programmes that are an integral part of a company's brand and corporate identity, including developing the infrastructure for managing their social investments that relate to children, youth, and families and providing strategic counsel in creating "win-win-win" business-related benefits for their employees, customers, and communities.

"Similarly, if many organisations experimenting with ISP initially approached these partnerships with a certain degree of trepidation-reflecting a lack of experience, misperception, and/or existing or past conflicts of interest-there is today a somewhat more nuanced understanding of the complexity of the motivations of each. For example, some in the NGO sector have considered corporate philanthropy to be solely motivated by a desire to improve a company's visibility and/or reputation.

However, in the same way corporations have come to understand how the social and economic development of potential customers and employees directly affect their bottom line, CSOs have in turn come to see areas of common purpose. So while recognising that certain motivations are, will and should remain distinct from sector to sector, globalisation has contributed to an expanding arena of common purpose.

POWER RELATIONS

An initial concern of many organisations-particularly CSOs-relates to real and/or perceived power asymmetries among the members of the partnership. Long-term studies on this particular dimension of ISPs could help shed light on the nature and degree of such asymmetries.

In addition to an examination of the more general question, it would be useful to have a number of organisation-specific studies that analyse whether their orientation, practices, objectives, style, etc. have shifted over time. The nature of the questions raised about ISP has evolved as experiences with these sorts of partnerships have grown. Much attention early on was concentrated on efforts to reach a common understanding of the term itself.

Many organisations, for example, struggled with long-standing skepticism or concern regarding the motivations of potential partners in the other sectors. Power asymmetries were a key concern, particularly on the part of some civil society actors who felt they would be compromised, co-opted or otherwise overwhelmed through close collaboration with government and/or business.

These concerns varied of course from country to country, from sector to sector, and from organisation to organisation, depending upon factors such as economic, political and historical context, the maturity of the sector and organisational strength.

Today, as civil society organisations gain greater confidence in what they have to offer a partnership, concern over power asymmetries has been reduced or, at least, has become more nuanced. CSOs recognise that government and business need them just as they need government and business.

Similarly, government and business representatives have come to recognise that their longstanding access to human, financial, and technical resources are today no match for the complexities of globalisation. As all three sectors become more experienced in crossing traditional sectoral boundaries, the issues that arise are at once strategic and practical.

Linking Grassroots Development

Another critical area for research is the connection between grassroots development and the legal, regulatory and policy environment at the national and international level. In a speech to the world leaders in attendance, Jean François Rischard, Vice President for Europe of the World Bank, urged the formation of Global Issues Networks. Rejecting the ability of existing organisations such as the Bank or the United Nations to resolve major, cross-cutting problems such as global warming for reasons having to do primarily with the need for speedy, decisive action, Rischard endorsed the idea of coalitions of governments, businesses, and NGOs organised to set international standards around issues of global concern.

GLOBALISATION AND ISP

Globalisation is a term that describes the reality of a world linked through instant communication, financial markets, and global responsibility. It provides enormous opportunity for commercial gain and an equally great responsibility to ensure that new resources are used to reduce existing inequities. There is no inherent value-negative or positive-to globalisation. The term describes the world in which we live. It poses new challenges and offers new solutions.

Different sectors in society have been encouraged to collaborate due to the decline in funding for international development, shifts in power from national governments to local entities, the growing involvement of the private sector in social issues, and the increasing number of capable civil society organisations. It was thought that ISP would strengthen individual organisations within each sector, offer a mechanism to resolve specific development issues, and lay the foundation for broader, systemic change.

12

PRINCIPLES AND PRACTICES OF MODERN PUBLIC RELATIONS

Public relations is now a recognised discipline around the world. It is an industry with millions of professionals who generally apply one basic theory of practice. It deals with the way we relate to our different audiences. There is a good way and a bad way to practice public relations. The Global Alliance is there to help with establishing world-wide guidance. Today, just about every private, public or social organisation, more or less consciously, uses public relations strategies, programmes and techniques. These strategies are implemented by developing and deploying communication tools and instruments that are designed to create and manage positive relationships with influential publics. We define influential publics as those believed capable of delaying or accelerating the pursued objectives of an organisation.

It is well documented in textbooks that this practice has been going on for more than a century in Anglo Saxon countries, some fifty years in the European continent and at least thirty years in a large part of the Rest of the World. As Marshall McCluhan's- the great Canadian whose vision of a global village is now a clear reality, and instantaneous -or zero time—communication continues to blanket our globe, we are constantly reminded that we need to adapt quickly to live and communicate in a world increasingly sans frontières (sem fronteiras) Clearly, this means that our outlook on life needs to be multidimensional to accommodate the diversity of races, countries, cultures, languages, that surround us. This becomes even more pertinent when we take into account the multiplicity of social, economic and political "divides" that tend to emphasise the disparities between east and west; north and south; black and white; developed and developing worlds; men and women; children and adults; teenagers and their parents.....so, how do we close the gap between these divides?

One of the solutions is to continue to segment our communication activities so that we have a consistent message that is tailored and more relevant to the segment of the population we are trying to reach. The days of 'one message fits all' are over. Yet too many of us continue to operate in this environment. First let's start with the fundamentals. There is an emerging world theory of public relations that is based on the concept of generic principles and specific applications.

The two-way symmetrical model is largely a model that organisations aspire to use. Just like Corporate social responsibility- CSR- two way symmetrical communication is not yet a reality in most organisations. Yet, as Dr. Grunig showed, it forms the basis of the characteristics of an excellent organisation. That is very much the 'aspirational' model for all professionals to follow. It is much more effective than the traditional 'push' method of communication because it adopts a mode of operation that focuses on listening and dialogue. Within this model of practice, the RACE formula-Research-Analysis-Communication and Evaluation stills forms the basis of our work.

The theory represents the generic aspect. The 'Specific Application' represents the manner in which the RACE formula produces a different set of tactical activities. So in theory two professionals from different countries can be tackling the same problem using the same theoretical framework, but because largely of context, they will choose different solutions.At its simplest form, public relations is a way to approach the way in which an organisation wants to relate to its many stakeholders. It is as much a specific discipline with its own body of knowledge and theories, than it is a management philosophy- particularly if the organisation has adopted the Corporate Social responsibility model of operation. But even if the organisation has not adopted CSR as a model, every time an organisation makes a decision, there are four broad sets of implications that require serious consideration.

Paul Holmes who writes an European PR newsletter describes it this way: Operational implications; financial implications; legal implications; and relationship or reputational implications. In most organisations, the first three sets of implications are considered routinely and formally at the highest level-there are senior executives whose responsibility it is to make sure those implications are clearly understood and fully incorporated into the decisionmaking process. Reputational implications, however, are often relegated to an afterthought. Rather than being asked for input when policy is being made, public relations people are too often called in after the fact to "spin" the selected policies, to make ill-considered decisions more palatable to a sceptical public.

Relationship implications should not override operational, financial, or legal concerns, they should be considered in tandem. This makes for a better decision. It is definitely not just an activity that supports a business line or a sub set of other activities that an organisation does. Most successful enterprises or large organisations have understood that to thrive and survive they must pay attention to their relationships with all of their contacts: employees, suppliers, clients, governments, lobby groups, etc. The Global Alliance estimates that in 2003 more than 3 million individuals were involved, in one way or another, in activities which may be defined as public relations, and it is possible to calculate, for that same year, the otherwise constantly growing annual economic impact of the profession is estimated at some 400 billion euro. Interestingly enough only a scant 10% of that 3 million are members of an institute or professional body.

If communication is the act of conveying ideas and information, and trust is such a fundamental issue in our global economy, then ethics is the glue that fosters a higher set of morals and principles by which we live. That is why, the public relations associations that form the Global Alliance have put some much emphasis over the years on ethics which culminated in the adoption of a universal code of ethics for the profession. For years our emphasis on ethics has gone unnoticed, now with Enron, Worldcom, Parmalat and others it gets the attention it deserves.

Here is a definition of Public relations that is close to universal: Public relations is the management, through communication, of perceptions and strategic relationships between an organisation and its internal and external stakeholders, for mutual benefit and a greater social order. Interestingly enough the Germans don't have a word for public relations. They call it: "Offentlichkeitsarbeit"and the meaning is: working in public, with the public, for the public. As you can see the German definition is much more oriented to the impact on the 'public sphere' and this is a very noble pursuit.

Two concepts of public relations are good public relations and poor public relations. Good public relations is focused on the long range—not on crises. Cumulative effects of public relations is like a savings account at the bank to which you make regular deposits and the interest compounds. It is about building relationships and when a crisis hits. Poor public relations is primarily focused on crisis, lack of a professional public relations programme, questionable ethics and a focus on short term goals. It may look and sound good, but doesn't last. Unfortunately poor public relations examples are all around us and have been around for a long time- 140 years ago, Abraham Lincoln delivered a speech in Bloomington, Illinois declaring "you may fool all the people some of the time; you can even fool some of the people all the time; but you can't fool all the people all of time". If he was referring to public relations- sure there was some good political rhetoric behind this quote, but he might have been thinking about it!

Most politicians at all levels and in all countries are quick to deplore the lack of public confidence or credibility in their own chosen profession. This is the same world-wide. Why have we lost faith in them?: Too much cynical use of short term tactics and too little professional public relations. They might win the battles with, evasive manoeuvres, deflection or Teflon answers, and propaganda—style campaigns. But they rarely win the war for public opinion.

Politicians are not alone suffering from a lack of trust. A 1996 extensive public survey on honesty in the workplace "Shades of Grey" conducted in the United States for PRSA found that:

— 61 % say that politicians make false promises (up 9% since 88)

— 51 % believe auto mechanics misinform or overcharge clients (up 16% since 88)

— 35% believe lawyers misinform or overcharge (up 18% since 88)

You might be asking yourself if other nations would do better in such a survey. Well, the CPRS in Canada commissioned an identical survey in 1997. The results of this survey of Canadians found that Canadians are only marginally more honest than our cousins to the south. The bottom line for public relations is that communicating credibility is tough and getting tougher. The public will discount what is said in any venue, by almost any medium by a considerable amount -- 30 to 50% of the message will be immediately discounted depending on the source and the context.

For example, the Shades of Gray study found that public expectations of truth and honesty from organisations was at 65%. So the people are not expecting the truth! and are discounting more than a third of what they hear ! Scary stuff ! especially if you are trying to convince someone your product or policy is better than the next guy's or your opponents! All the more reason to practice good public relations and avoid the pitfalls of manipulation and disinformation.

But how do we get out of this quagmire? By making conscious choices to GROW trust. Without trust from within the organisation, and externally, no business strategy is going to be as effective as it otherwise could. It requires putting programmes in place that demonstrate behaviorally not rhetorically that an organisation has concern for its employees, suppliers and external audiences or clients. Actions have always spoken louder than words. And coincidently, growing trust is almost always a key public relations objective. Effective public relations starts with understanding and listening. It is rooted in complete transparency and open and frank discussion of the issues. We know that public relations works well in the following areas:

— Formation of attitudes or opinions; in other words:

— education;

— persuasion or changing perceptions and opinions; and

— changing behaviors.

We do know that public relations works most effectively when it is approached strategically, systematically and consistently. You can't do "a little public relations" and expect a lot of results. The impact of public relations builds over time, with repetition of key strategic messages in a variety of contexts. That, is using the force, the power of public relations. These good examples are not always splashy and visible—but they are highly effective and long lasting, and if they are visible the effect is even more lasting. This is important for everyone, whether your business is large or small, highly visible or less visible. Client satisfaction surveys, feedback lines, speeches, community sponsorships...these are the often the less splashy activities of a good public relations programme. Of course a good advertising programme never hurts.

It is always a good thing to incorporate long range and short range goals. The idea is to open channels of communications with your stakeholders, talk about their issues, inform them, influence them when they are ready to listen, Before their minds are made up. Think of sponsoring a community programme, conduct customer satisfaction surveys, have open houses and workshops about your trade. You will be surprised at the results. Public relations is sometimes referred to as "smoke and mirrors". But only by those who have never experienced its positive results, or who have run into incompetent practitioners.

Let us first consider what public relations will not do: It will not make up for deficiencies in your product and customer service operation. Although in a crisis good public relations may reduce the negative impact, bad public relations can make matters worse. Public relations is not a substitute for corporate planning, nor can it turn a slack sales force into record-breaking superstars. Also, contrary to popular misconception, it will not create a positive image of a company that is poorly run, is a bad neighbor, or has serious ethical and funding problems. That being said, this is what public relations will do:

It will target and educate your market's information gatekeepers—the analysts and the media—about your product or your position on an issue. They, in turn, will tell others about your company. This will crystallise public opinion in your favor. It can maintain the satisfaction of your customers, generate sales leads, enhance your reputation in the community, and help you to attract top flight employees. As you can see these examples have nothing to do with crises and media flare-ups but are just as powerful when handled professionally and with continuity.

Good public relations is a balance between listening and talking. Understanding this fundamental premise is the foundation of powerful public relations. Good public relations advice is like good weather forecasts. The power comes from the positioning of the function as advisory to senior management. Remember how a public event or a crisis can make or break you. Remember that public opinion is about perceptions. Some organisations have understood and indeed demanded from their public relations staff that they play the role of public or devil's advocate. These lucky practitioners are required to listen to other voices, perform a reality check on management, and play devil's advocate with senior managers. Organisations don't need "yes people". They need public relations staff who are not afraid to speak their minds, and to go against established positions. Credibility and trust are the most important assets an organisation has working for it. Public relations' first priority is to build and maintain this credibility as you would with a bank account, the more deposits you make, the bigger cushion you will have when a rainy day comes.

Those organisations which include public relations at the management table expect their public relations practitioners to understand the management problems, while at the same time relaying to management the concepts and activities that they will not hear from the other professional advisors. Things like public opinion research, town hall meetings, interviews with influential reporters, meeting community groups, resolving differences and resisting the urge to crush all opposing points of view. Public relations people are change agents. But we must remember the human side of change. People don't mind change, they just mind being changed in their ways- it doesn't just happen, you have to introduce change. Grasping this important nuance puts you in the proper perspective to achieve powerful public relations.

The influence of Public relations goes beyond cleaning up the image of an organisation—it's a job of guiding the organisation on how to manage all relationships with stakeholders—and that's not just communicating—it's also acting better and trying to achieve some harmony. There can only be harmony if there is effective dialogue and dialogue is always a key objective in public relations. We either try to establish it, reinforce it or engage different groups in dialogue. In a small way organisations like the Global Alliance are doing their part, by stressing commonality rather than differences; collaboration rather than conflict as we unite the profession world-wide.

Some of the practitioners believe that through the work of the Global Alliance, and in particular its Global Protocol on Ethics , public relations practitioners, through their national associations, will have the tools to promote good governance through truth, respect and responsibility, in other words, through ethical, as well as effective communication. This protocol requires each practitioner to pledge:

To conduct ourselves professionally, with integrity, truth, accuracy, fairness, and responsibility to our clients, our client publics, and to an informed society to improve our individual competence and advance the knowledge and proficiency of the profession through continuing education and research and where available, through the pursuit of professional accreditation. To adhere to the principles of the Universal Code of Professional Standards for the Practice of Public Relations. In most advanced democracies, these recent years have witnessed an unprecedented number of new regulations or self imposed constraints in an effort to set norms to the right of organisations to express themselves in the public arena and the public policy process.

The Global Alliance has writen a report on the state of hard regulations- legislated solutions- and soft regulations—voluntary or policy driven solutions—on the PR industry by eaxmining in detail three countries. Although full regulation of the public relations profession per se is largely absent today -save for excpetions such as the countries of Nigeria, Panama and Brazil- many of the profession's operative practices are increasingly being regulated, particularly those which have a stronger impact on the public interest: political public relations, lobbying, public sector and social public relations, health communication, financial pr, consumer pr. This trend is happening country by country, in a totally unharmonised fashion, either with the introduction of hard laws approved by national parliaments or by soft laws introduced by regulatory authorities or by other self regulating bodies.

This regulatory growth is such that, unlike in the 70's, 80's and 90's when, for example in the USA, only the legendary figure of Edward Bernays stubbornly advocated the full regulation/licensing of public relations while the rest of the professional community rhetorically invoked 'freedom of expression' and 'right to bear grievance'....respectively the first and the fifth amendment of the US Constitution- some respected figures of the professional community today are beginning to have second thoughts and wonder if a full regulation of the profession would not be a more effective as well as 'elegant' way to reassure the public interest of the fundamentally democratic raison d'etre of public relations while, at the same time, protecting the profession's overall tumbling reputation.

Of course it needs to be perfectly clear and understood, at least from professionals who have a thorough knowledge of the ups and downs of regulation because it's part of their day-to-day activity, that it is not simply a law which will change behaviours at large, and that the very policing of such law would be a highly complex matter, as at least in the three license-mandatory countries indicated above there seems to have been little if any effect on the dayto-day professional practice: it is sufficient for professionals to call themselves communicators or something else rather than public relators to avoid compliance with the law.... However it would make a great difference within a professional community to be able to publicly 'call foul' if someone, even a non member, committed a criminal offense because a universal regulation was violated, rather than balking, as is the more frequent case today, in the fear of being sued for libel every time. We are too often silent on matters within our own backwyard.

We can now see very clearly is the proliferation of pervasive communication channels. These are beginning to have a potentially detrimental impact on individuals. With everyone empowered 'to have a voice' the competition to be heard has the effect of diminishing individual attention and concentration capabilities—evidenced by one recent study which purports that in 2003 each human-being received and distributed 800 million bytes of information. The recent phenomenon of blogging is a case in point. Now everyone who has something to say can set up a blog and let people read their thoughts on everything under the sun. Of course it did not take long for specialisation to take hold here and we now have several blogs about PR.

Then there is the CSR- Corporate Social Responsibility trend. An entire cottage industry supports this new dogma of management. The United nations has adopted a Global Compact as a way to guide governance issues. This CSR phenomenon has accelerated awareness within the public relations community of today's most reputed theoretical approach to the profession—the Grunig model- which in 2004 marks its 20th anniversary as a framework theory by which public relations is taught/ understood.

Another trend that is the increased interest in accreditation- or professional certification programmes. Now that certified education programmes, the idea that individuals should obtain a professional credential-like the APR which is in use in at least nine countries around the world- is gaining ground. The Global Alliance has decide to explore the creation of its second world- class standard in the area of professional certification. A benchmarking process is now underway to determine how much commonality we have between the various accreditation regimes. Professional associations are there to help practitioners get better by offering conferences like this one and other workshops, knowledge as well as to offer a network of contacts. Above all, these institutions are there to promote professionalism and standards in our industry. Employers need qualified, ethically minded and preferably accredited professionals who take their profession seriously on their staff.

Public relations is part art, part science. It is up to public relations professional to use the power of listening, to find out what the public is thinking and relay that to management, formulate a public relations programme.

BIBLIOGRAPHY

Baskin, Otis & Arnoff, Craig, (1992) *Public Relations: The Profession and The Practice*, 3rd ed, Brown & Benchmark.

Broom, Glen M.& Dozier, David M, (1989) *Using Research in Public Relations: Applications to Program Management*, Prentice-Hall.

Cutlip, Scott & Center, Allen, (1994) *Effective Public Relations*, 7th ed. Prentice Hall .

Cutlip, Scott, (1995) *Public Relations History: From the Seventeenth to the Twentieth Century*, L. Erlbaum

Deighton, J, (1996). "The Future of Interactive Marketing", *Harvard Business Review*, November-December: 151-162

Ellsworth, J.H. & Ellsworth, M.V, (1995) *Marketing on the Internet*. New York: John Wiley & Sons. Inc.

Fisher, J, (1998) "*Future Trends*", In Lawrence, E.; Corbitt, B. Tidwell, A.; Fisher, J.; Lawrence, J.R. Internet Commerce: Digital Models for Business. Miton Qld: John Wiley & Sons

Fitzgerald, S.S. & Spagnolia, N, (1999) "Four Predictions for PR Practitioners in the New Millenium", *Public Relations Quarterly*, Precision Public Relations. NY & London: Longman Inc.

Freedman, D.H, (1992) "Is management still a science"? *Harvard Business Review*, Vol 70 (Nov-Dec): 26-28

Grunig, James & Hunt, Todd, (1984) *Managing Public Relations*, HBJ College

Harris, T.L, (1998) "*Value-Added Public Relations: The Secret Weapon of Integrated Marketing*". NTC Business Books. Illinois Harrison, S. 1995.

Howard, C.M, (1998) *How your Employee Communications Programs Can Boost Productivity and Pride,* Public Relations Quarterly, Fall 1998. 43(3): 15-23

Hunt, T. & Grunig, J.E, (1994) "*Public Relations Techniques*", Forth Worth: Harcourt Brace College Publishers.

Lesly, Philip, (1991) Lesly's Handbook of Public Relations and Communications. AMACOM.

White, C., Raman, N, (1999) "*The World Wide Web as a Public Relations Medium: The Use of Research, Planning, and Evaluation in Site Development*". Public Relations Review. Vol 25(4): 405-419 White, J; Mazur, L.1995.

INDEX

INDEX